"This intensely contemporary book defends a subversive idea: *primary erotogenic masochism* constitutes the *nucleus* of our ego, an early stage where Eros and Thanatos join forces and embrace. To convince ourselves of this, it was necessary to appropriate *what is beyond the pleasure principle*, to prove that the analytical session is 'an act of the flesh', to imbibe literature and cinema, to philosophize with Tertullian, Spinoza and Hannah Arendt, to take as a 'patient' the fictional character of a Nazi officer, or a journalistic investigation into the war in Rwanda, albeit not without revealing our organic intimacy as psychoanalysts. Some try, not enough, not really, but Marilia Aisenstein has done it with writing that is as rigorous as it is vibrant."

Julia Kristeva, *psychoanalyst, essayist, novelist and Professor Emeritus of the University of Paris*

"This is a remarkable and needed book, not only for psychoanalysts but also for all those interested in better understanding how the human mind works. Marilia Aisenstein is one of our main psychoanalytic thinkers, and she shows masterfully how to blend theory, clinical examples and different expressions of culture. The presence of primal masochism and its different levels is central to human existence, and it can lead us to the sublime as well as to the horror. I strongly recommend this book. Aisenstein conducts us with elegance and erudition through the labyrinths of pain till the pleasure of thinking and thus feeling alive."

Cláudio Laks Eizirik, *training and supervising analyst, Porto Alegre Psychoanalytic Society, Professor Emeritus of Psychiatry, Former President of IPA*

Desire, Pain and Thought

Desire, Pain and Thought presents a new perspective on primal erotogenic masochism, which Marilia Aisenstein regards as the core of psychoanalytic theory.

Aisenstein distinguishes between pathological masochism – the active search for pain – and primal erotogenic masochism, which she believes develops in early childhood. *Desire, Pain and Thought* explains that the formation of this response in a child is essential to the survival of the individual and the development of resilience. Aisenstein skilfully and convincingly uses her deep understanding of metapsychology and her mastery of Freud's seminal papers to demonstrate that thought is one of the manifestations of desire which implies a painful renunciation of the object of desire. By moving away from its pathological, negative connotation to a more positive one, the book presents an understanding of masochism as "the guardian of life".

Desire, Pain and Thought will be essential reading for psychoanalysts in practice and in training.

Marilia Aisenstein is a training and supervising psychoanalyst of the Hellenic Psychoanalytical Society and the Paris Psychoanalytic Society. She is a former president of the Paris Society and of the Paris Psychosomatic Institute and editor and co-founder of the *French Review of Psychosomatics*. She has written both chapters and books, mainly on psychosomatics and hypochondria, transference, pain and destructiveness, and over 150 papers in French, Greek and English, which have been translated into Spanish, German and Portuguese. She received the Maurice Bouvet Award in 1992.

Psychoanalytic Ideas and Applications Series
Series Editor: Silvia Flechner

IPA Publications Committee Fred Busch, Natacha Delgado, Nergis Güleç, Thomas Marcacci, Carlos Moguillansky, Rafael Mondrzak, Angela M. Vuotto, Gabriela Legoretta (consultant)

For more information about this series, please visit: www.routledge.com

Desire, Pain and Thought

Primal Masochism and
Psychoanalytic Theory

Marilia Aisenstein

Translated by Andrew Weller

Routledge
Taylor & Francis Group
LONDON AND NEW YORK

Designed cover image: © Getty Images

First published in English 2023
by Routledge
4 Park Square, Milton Park, Abingdon, Oxon OX14 4RN

and by Routledge
605 Third Avenue, New York, NY 10158

Routledge is an imprint of the Taylor & Francis Group, an informa business

© 2023 Marilia Aisenstein

Translated by Andrew Weller

Published in French by Editions d'Ithaque, Paris 2020

British Library Cataloguing-in-Publication Data
A catalogue record for this book is available from the British Library

ISBN: 978-1-032-05462-9 (hbk)
ISBN: 978-1-032-05464-3 (pbk)
ISBN: 978-1-003-19765-2 (ebk)

DOI: 10.4324/9781003197652

Typeset in Palatino
by Apex CoVantage, LLC

To Paul Averoff, my beloved grandson

Contents

Series editor's foreword

Desire, Pain and Thought

The Publications Committee of the International Psychoanalytic Association continues, with the present volume, the series "Psychoanalytic Ideas and Applications".

The aim of this series is to focus on the scientific production of significant authors, whose works are outstanding contributions to the development of the psychoanalytic field and to set out relevant ideas and themes, generated during the history of psychoanalysis, that deserve to be known and discussed by present day psychoanalysts.

The relationship between psychoanalytic ideas and their applications needs to be put forward from the perspective of theory, clinical practice and research, in order to maintain their validity for contemporary psychoanalysis.

The Publication's Committee's objective is to share these ideas with the psychoanalytic community and with professionals in other related disciplines, so as to expand their knowledge and generate a productive interchange between the text and the reader.

The IPA Publications Committee is pleased to publish the English translation of Marilia Aisenstein's book *Desire, Pain and Thought*, which was first published in French in October 2020. The Publications Committee has already published two of Marilia Aisenstein's books: *Psychosomatics Today* and *Psychosomatic Today revisited Edition*, which have elicited much interest in the psychanalytic community.

Marilia's Aisenstein's main goal in this book is to expose her views on primal erotogenic masochism, which she sees as the core of psychoanalytic theory. The book provides an original contribution to the topic of masochism which moves away from its pathological and negative connotation to a more positive one in which masochism could be thought of as "the guardian of life". As she states, "without it we would commit suicide at the first disappointment". She does, however, differentiate pathological masochism, which is the active search for pain, from the primal erotogenic masochism, which she believes develops at a very early stage, when a "masochistic nucleus of the ego" is formed in the child, which, in her view, will be essential to ensure the survival of the individual and the development of resilience.

The table of contents allows the reader to appreciate the richness of the content of the book, as one can value the different angles from which the author studies and reflects on the notion of erotogenic masochism. There are chapters titled "the enigma of pain", "the birth of desire", "the absence of masochism", "the notion of thinking and the destruction of thinking", to name a few. It is impressive, the way in which the author creatively links together the notions of desire, pain and thought. She skilfully and convincingly uses her deep understanding of metapsychology and her mastery of Freud's seminal papers to demonstrate that thought is one of the manifestations of desire, which, by definition, implies a painful renunciation of the object of desire. She explains the trajectory involved in the transformation of a human need into the desire of an object and the development of the capacity to tolerate pain which is intrinsic to the absence of the object of desire. Using her own words, the author states, "only desire can give rise to the activity of thought, the inalienable pleasure and privilege of man". She develops this idea further by stating that thinking is not only painful but sometimes dangerous, because to think is to exist as a subject, to differentiate oneself from others, with all the risks associated with it. The author presents clinical cases that illuminate in a brilliant and clear manner the theoretical elaborations she puts forward. Moreover, the author has a beautiful and clear writing style that captures the interest of the reader. She has the ability to write complex ideas in a captivating manner. It is a pleasure to read.

This book is an important contribution to the study of masochism by a much-appreciated and well-known author. It will be of much interest and help from both theoretical and clinical perspectives to psychoanalysts and to clinicians with a psychoanalytic approach. One should be thankful to Dr. Aisenstein for this exceptional work that has made this volume possible for the English readership.

Gabriela Legorreta
Series Editor
Chair, IPA Publications Committee

Foreward

A user guide

In order to help readers find their way into this very rich book and to gain access to its depth and gravity, I suggest that:

(1) *They let themselves be "passively" impregnated* by Marilia Aisenstein's thinking, by its rigour, associated with the freedom and sensuality of her writing, to which her many literary references bear witness. Blending, perhaps it would be better to say associating, is a decisive operation for this reflection which likes to conciliate contrary and divergent points of view (philosophical, psychoanalytic, poetic) in order to reveal the unique common foundation; for example, the view of death that the author develops, albeit solidly grounded in the Freudian tradition of the drives, proves on reading to be close to Rilke's poetic meditation, making death the centre of life. This naturally requires a free-floating reading of this extremely dense text which reveals under the manifest content its latent content. I am personally grateful to Marilia for having drawn my attention to the proximity of thought linking Freud and Rilke. In "The Book of Poverty and Death" (1903), the latter writes:

> O Lord, give each of us our own death:
>   A dying that is born of each life,
> Our own desire, our purpose, love, dearth.
>
> For we are only rind of fruit, and leaf.
> The great death, which each of us contains,
> Is that fruit round which the world turns.
>   (Rilke, 2008, p. 163, 165)

In the author's language, the *"great death"* becomes "primary erotogenic masochism" which, as the present book continually hammers home, is the essence of favourable psychic activity. Admittedly, poetic elegance is replaced here by a certain roughness of scientific discourse, which is necessary for the psychotherapeutic application of this discovery.

(2) *They let themselves be impregnated by what it shows* about how the author listens to her patients, listening to herself while listening to the other person. Most of the clinical cases presented follow this thread: this gives rise to fascinating narratives that draw the reader into the intimacy of analysis and towards the heart of the creation of the inner discourse of the analyst; furthermore, it leads the author, as it were incidentally, to offer quite a unique reflection on the "organic" solidarity of the transference and the countertransference.

(3) *They discover how she appropriates*, in the strong sense of the term, Freudian thought, how she makes it her own, transforms it, and thereby saves it from the strictly "academic" and thus doctrinal fate of fetishisation. It is the right and duty of every analyst to build his or her own theory and then to present it when he or she has acquired the certainty that it can fortify his or her colleagues in the hard task that has fallen upon them. Hence, the author's reflections, which enrich the Freudian heritage, in particular, on the negative figures of death, pain, a certain representation of the feminine and the work of eroticising waiting and frustration. This erotisation turns unpleasure into pleasure and thereby contributes to the establishment of a stable pleasure principle, clearly turned towards reality and conservation. She is able to make these advances due to a close reading of Freud's work, whose errings and triumphs she shares with us: "The masochistic pleasure of pain becomes in the second drive theory the very model of pleasure", she writes (p. 36).

(4) *They convince themselves that these theoretical advances* must be received with great openness of mind and that they can in no case give rise to an overly intellectual scientific debate; for they are not so much important in themselves as signs of displacements accomplished by the analyst between what he or she has inherited and what he or she has done with them. "Why", she asks, "do we have a liking for one kind of metapsychology rather than another?" The answer is given without ambiguity: because, while our scientific destinies depend in part on a reasoned choice, they always, and first and foremost, manifest the inspirational force of our filiations. In this book, Marilia Aisenstein presents the mentors who traced the new path that she adopted: Benno Rosenberg, Michel Fain and André Green, all enriched as much by their common fidelity to Freud as by their independence from him and between themselves; and regarding the philosophical part of her inspiration, Tertullian, and even Cicero. The author thus makes room for all those who have inspired her or those whom she has admired, "whether they believed in God or not".

* * *

The analyst does not work with his thoughts alone, but with his being as it has been changed, "transformed" – I like Bion's strong term – by his theoretical reflection. Thought must become in him, as our author writes with no less force, an "act of the flesh". Freud (1917) took the measure of this when, right in the middle of the text "Mourning and melancholia", he conjures up, as if in a hallucination, the figure of Hamlet – his double – who recites the monologue beginning with *To be or not to be*. Why, he asks himself, faced with the diminution of self-regard to which the hero exposes himself, "does a man have to be ill before he can be accessible to a truth of this kind?" (p. 246).

There can be no doubt that anyone who expresses in front of others such a lack of self-regard, like Prince Hamlet, is ill, whether he is telling the truth or whether he is doing himself an injustice, more or less.

And Freud discovered, by means of this psychodramatic method of an incarnation that had nothing conceptual about it, the price of madness that has to be paid for lucidity!

Even if the guiding thread of the author's reflections is primary erotogenic masochism, as it grounds subjectivity by calling pain to the rescue, or what Michel Fain called "pleasant passivity", which protects the subject from the alienation of phallic narcissism, or as it brings into play the blending of the life and death drives – whether it is blending or an alliance – this challenge overlaps, at all the levels of the author's thought, with many other themes, which radiate out from it yet are more clinical. Among the themes discussed are: female psychology (the heroic fatigue of women); negation, which "is not a refusal but the root of being"; religion, drawing its source in guilt; and the extreme operations of de-subjectivisation and de-objectalisation that André Green saw at work in the heavy pathologies of psychosis and borderline states and that Marilia Aisenstein, in a poignant moment of her book, denounces as being the source of all barbarism. A preface is not a survey; I simply want to highlight the arborescence of this thought.

Apart from the fact that it is a solid scientific reflection, well-argued and convincing, this text is a lesson of life; the writing is, as it were, enchanted, showing everything that literature and psychoanalysis can offer man in his suffering, his moroseness or unhappiness; it shows how pain is a salutary weapon when primal masochism makes it gain access to the status of pleasure. I have never heard anyone speak so simply and with such clarity about pain: as the author convinces us, we must not seek its raison d'être, but rather accept it as a fact, as material from which the mind first distils desire, and then thought.

Whatever meaning we attribute to the three words that comprise the title, we will be persuaded, after reading the book, that they are but one, and that, in this blending, they are the very definition of what the author calls the "act of the flesh". And, to my great relief, I finally understand that this semantic constellation discovered by our author expresses the matter so much better than the Freudian term – scientific, certainly, but very bar-baric – of anti-cathexis was meant to imply: namely, that the specifically painful turning round upon the self by the primal ego of attention and the libido, which are normally turned towards the external world and its object, is sometimes salvatory.

The quality that Jean Laplanche requires of any analytic theory applies perfectly to this resolutely modern theorisation. We must suppose that analytic theory, at its most general level, should show us how, in what conditions, and with what results and failures, and at what price the subject "theorises" and metabolises the enigmas with which interhuman intercommunication faces him. In a certain way, analytic theory is thus a metatheory, compared with the fundamental theorisation operated by the human being: in the first place, this is not in order to appropriate nature but to bind anxiety in relation to the trauma of the enigma.

J.C. Rolland
April 2020

References

Freud, S. (1917 [1915]). *Mourning and Melancholia. S.E.*, 14. London: Hogarth, pp. 243–258.

Rilke, M. (2008/1918). The Book of Poverty and Death. In: *The Book of Hours*, ed. Ben Hutchinson, trans. Susan Ranson. Rochester, NY: Camden House, pp. 156–197.

Introduction

Primal masochism: the navel of psychoanalytic theory

I have long been interested in the Freudian conception of primal eroto-genic masochism, described by Freud (1924) in "The economic problem of masochism", a text I have always found deeply moving. We can see Freud asking himself: is it possible that pain is tinged with pleasure? Worse: is it possible that pain and the search for pain govern psychic life? But what, then, becomes of the "pleasure principle"? These questions were crucial and remain so today.

I had the great pleasure and opportunity of working with Michel Fain, as well as with Bruno Rosenberg, who was not only a mentor for me but also a true friend. When I was writing my book on Fain (Aisenstein, 2000), he was kind enough to offer me an unpublished article to include in it, and on that very day, he gave it the title: "A propos du masochisme érogène primaire. Dialogue imaginaire avec Bruno Rosenberg" (ibid, pp 65–71)[1] – "imaginary" because Benno was already ill and was to pass away prematurely in 2003.

In this article, Fain evokes the clinical situation of those patients in whom, he says, "bad over-exciting conditions have prevented pleasant passivity from establishing itself. All that is registered in the mind is the lack of this experience. In such cases, only activity is valued, and phallic narcissism will infiltrate the ego-ideal" (ibid., p. 71). Further on, he continues: "It was these observations, in most cases in connection with somatic patients, that led me to speak of 'incomplete' masochism. The 'incompleteness' pertains to the passive position rendered inaccessible by early traumatic experiences" (ibid.).

I think it is worth reflecting on this text, which precedes by one year "Mentalisation et passivité", the very last article by Fain (2001), which was published in the *Revue française de psychosomatique*. The notion of an "incompleteness of masochism pertaining to the passive position" is original and very illustrative of the thought of Michel Fain, who, during supervisions, always drew our attention to what was missing: "Think about what is, and what is beneath the surface", he would say to us.

The notion of "incomplete masochism" (Fain) or the "incompletion of primary masochism" (my term) is at the intersection between the

DOI: 10.4324/9781003197652-1

psychoanalysis of the neuroses, psychoses and borderline states, and the psychoanalysis of somatising patients.

"Here we are once more confronted with the accursed problem of masochism!", exclaimed Ferenczi in 1931. And in the introduction of the collective book *L'Enigme du masochisme*, Jacques André (2000) wrote, "There is enough there to upset theory and lead analysts to say anything: pleasure in displeasure, for example. The pitfalls to practice are no less daunting, and the trap becomes unavoidable, if suffering, instead of acting as the motor of progress in the treatment, become its desired end" (p. 1).

In two texts, "The problem of the acceptance of unpleasant ideas" (1926) and "On the acceptance of unpleasure" (1932), Ferenczi deals with the question of *pleasant passivity* that was later studied by Fain.

* * *

"Why do we have a liking for one kind of metapsychology rather than another?"

Freud, an outstanding genius, left us a corpus that remains the basis of all psychoanalytic thought. André Green remained authentically Freudian, while deriving all the consequences from Freud's work. He chose the axis that leads from negative narcissism to de-objectalisation, de-subjectivisation, negative hallucination and blank psychosis, and also left us an oeuvre in the full sense of the term. In this book, my imaginary interlocutors are primarily Michel Fain and Benno Rosenberg.

As a child, I wanted to understand what thought consisted of. I was convinced that only headaches led to important and interesting ideas. This kind of questioning led me to undertake studies in philosophy. And yet it was only much later on that I acknowledged that the question of masochism represented for me the *navel of psychoanalytic theory*. In my opinion, our theories, whether implicit or explicit, are deeply personal and indispensable for thinking about clinical work.

When I was still very young, I saw both psychotic patients in the context of the Mental Health Association in the 13th area of Paris (ASM13) and somatic patients at the Institute of Psychosomatics (IPSO). They were exciting days. Together with Jacques Azoulay, Victor Souffir, Josiane Chambrier and Domonique Deyon, we saw psychotic patients or families, and we set up an exploratory psychodrama led by Benno Rosenberg.

One day, when we were having lunch in the refectory, I asked Benno about the origin of his interest in masochism. He told me the following story: his father had been a professor and head of internal medicine in Bucharest during the rise of Nazism, but he was banished by anti-Semitic laws to a little village, where he replaced a retired country doctor. The peasant women that he treated remained mistrustful, and one of them told him one day: "With the old doctor it hurt. His injections, his bandages, all his treatments were painful, and that was why they were effective".

These women could not have confidence in a doctor whose injections were painless.

This story is paradigmatic of a belief or unconscious fantasy rooted in the psyche, according to which physical or mental suffering is a price human beings have to pay for their lives. It is an absurd belief for a rational mind, but the Christian religion seized upon it to erect its theory of original sin, paradise lost and redemptive suffering.

If Freud, who had tackled the phenomenon of primal masochism as early as 1905 in his *Three Essays on the Theory of Sexuality* (Freud, 1905), took almost twenty years to recognise, painfully, its existence in 1924, it was no doubt on account of the incongruous aspect for scientific thought of "religious" belief. Yet it is the psyche of man that "invented" religion in order to give credibility to fantasies and beliefs that were scarcely convincing in themselves.

Masochism is a "guardian of life"; without it, we would commit suicide when faced with the first major disappointment. It enables us to stand firm and to hope. It is because of it that man is able to survive and resist the most tragic and extreme conditions such as wars of religion and genocides, when the barbarity of man, the most inhuman of the animals, is unleashed. And yet, in everyday vocabulary, masochism has bad press. Calling someone a "masochist" is insulting.

I hope to persuade my readers, whether or not they are my psychoanalytic colleagues, that this is an error. Anyone who appears to be seeking suffering is suffering, in fact, from a *lack* of primary erotogenic masochism.

The clinical phenomenon of masochism existed before psychoanalysis, with the exception of sexual masochism, which I will not be discussing because its manifestations are the same as those of secondary masochism, also called "moral masochism".

The need for punishment, the quest for failure and excessive guilt have always been present in literature, ever since antiquity. Formerly, psychiatrists called the quest for pain, whether suffered or inflicted, *algolagnia*.

For Freud, as early as 1905, three forms of masochism could be distinguished: erotogenic, feminine and moral. The first, the pleasure of sexual excitation, is at the basis of the two others. Feminine masochism does not specifically concern women and is known through male fantasies; it concerns psychic bisexuality. Moral masochism is revealed by forms of behaviour dictated by unconscious guilt.

For me, these behaviours, or symptoms, are the epiphenomenon of a failure of the primary erotogenic masochism which binds the drives, described by Freud (1924) in "The economic problem of masochism", which is the subject of this book. I will come back to it in several chapters. This primary erotogenic masochism is the vestige of, and witness to, a phase of formation where there is a mixture of the two drives: Eros and the death drive.

It could only be conceived within the second drive theory. It concerns a very early stage, like primary narcissism, when a "masochistic nucleus of the ego" is formed in the child, which, in my opinion, will ensure his survival and his resilience.

The term "resilience" is not a metapsychological concept. It is, above all, used by Boris Cyrulnik.[2] Yet, in my view, he correctly describes the effects of the masochistic nucleus of the ego.

I have chosen here to leave aside perverse sexual masochism (see Nacht, 1938), which is better known than the other forms; it was the subject of a treatise by Richard von Krafft-Ebing (1840–1902). A contemporary of Freud, he was the one who created the term "masochism". In his *Psychopathia Sexualis* (Krafft-Ebing, 1886), he brought together under the term "masochism" all the clinical manifestations of sexual masochism, concerning which he curiously made a "pathological magnification of the female psychic elements".[3]

This is an opportunity to mention the figure of Leopold von Sacher-Masoch: a scholar with an enlightened mind, a journalist and professor at the University of Graz, he was the first to campaign for young women to be accepted at faculties in Austria. Born in 1836, he was very well-known in his life time, famous throughout Europe for his novels, tales and short stories, as well as for his modernist, anti-conformist and anti-nationalist positions. He received the Legion of Honour in 1886. After his death in 1895, his work was forgotten and his books burned under the regime of Nazi Germany. It was not until the 1960s, and in particular the preface by Gilles Deleuze to "Venus in Furs" (Sacher-Masoch, 1870), that this writer was talked about again. In 2004, some of his writings appeared in French, *The Love of Plato, Diderot in St Petersburg* and *An Insane Testament;* while *Tales of the Ghetto, The Enemy of Women, Jewish Tales and Little Russians, Between Two Windows and Lemberg's Black Cabinet* were published in German.

I want to do justice here to this author who was handled roughly and remained marginal.

Among other fictionalised stories, Sacher-Masoch had published "Venus in Furs" in 1870, which the dreadful psychiatrist Richard Krafft-Ebing, an ancestor of modern sexology, made use of to illustrate sexual masochism. The author had to fight for many years to see to it that his family name did not remain associated with a perversion, and it would seem that he took Krafft-Ebing to court several times, winning his case each time, even if it is still true that he lost the battle.

To conclude these introductory thoughts, I would like to stress that clinical masochism in its moral form, in particular, in the "negative therapeutic reaction", led to many clinical failures, which led Freud to reconsider his first drive theory. The recognition of the role of erotogenic masochism in binding the drives was to be the consequence of this necessary revision.

Notes

1 This text had not been published hitherto: it is included here in the annexes at the end of the book.

2 See Cyrulnik (1999) *Un Merveilleux malheur*, in which the author reflects on the processes of self-reparation invented by the survivors of the Holocaust. In *Les Vilains Petits Canards* (Cyrulnik, 2000), he shows how these processes are set up in the very first days of life and make resistance and reconstruction possible.
3 On perverse masochism, see the very interesting article by Michel de M'Uzan (1972).

References

Aisenstein, M. (2000). *Michel Fain*. Paris: Presses Universitaires de France, coll. "Psychanalystes d'aujourd'hui".

André, J. (Ed.). (2000). *L'enigme du masochisme*. Paris: Presses Universitaires de France.

Cyrulnik, B. (1999). *Un Merveilleux malheur*. Paris: Odile Jacob.

Cyrulnik, B. (2000). *Les Vilains Petits Canards*. Paris: Odile Jacob.

Fain, M. (2001). Mentalisation et passivité. *Revue française de psychosomatique* 1(19): 29–37.

Ferenczi, S. (1926/1950). The problem of the acceptance of unpleasant ideas: Advances in the knowledge of the sense of reality. In: *Further Contributions to the Theory and Technique of Psychoanalysis*. London: Hogarth, pp. 366–379.

Ferenczi, S. (1932/1988). On the acceptance of unpleasure. In: *The Clinical Diary of Sándor Ferenczi*, ed. Judith Dupont. Cambridge, MA: Harvard University Press, pp. 31–34.

Freud, S. (1905). *Three Essays on the Theory of Sexuality*. S.E., 7. London: Hogarth, pp. 123–243.

Freud, S. (1924). The economic problem of masochism. S.E., 19. London: Hogarth, pp. 155–170.

Krafft-Ebing, R. von (1886/1894). *Psychopathia Sexualis*, trans. R Krafft-Ebing & C. G. Chaddock. Philadelphia: F.A. Davis Company.

M'Uzan, M. de (1972). Un cas de masochisme pervers, esquisse d'une théorie. In: *De l'art à la mort*. Paris: Gallimard.

Nacht, S. (1938). Le masochisme. *Revue française de psychanalyse* 10(2): 171–291. Available on https://gallica.bnf.fr/ark:/12148/bpt6k11O117q.r=langfr.f170. pagination.

Sacher-Masoch, L. von (1870). Venus in Furs. In: *Masochism: Coldness and Cruelty & Venus in Furs*, eds. G. Deleuze, L. Sacher-Masoch. New York, NY: Zone Books, 1989, pp. 143–171.

1 The enigma of pain*

Sulphurous Japanese writer Tanizaki places in the mouth of a man who had lost his virility in the Hiroshima disaster a testamentary request in which he asks his unfaithful young wife to attend his suicide, which he has planned to last for several hours and to be very painful.

In a letter dated 1953, Imazato Masukichi, the hero of this story, expresses his last wishes: he wants her to be present, seated opposite him and never take her eyes off him. He adds that it was out of love for her and in order to ensure her happiness that he had made this irrevocable decision in complete freedom.

This letter is an extract from *Chroniques inhumaines* (Inhuman Chronicles) (Tanizaki, 1997–1998), a novel by the Japanese writer Jun'ichirō Tanizaki [1886–1965] In the pages that follow it, the author reconstitutes the history of Masukichi, whom we see injured, lost and wandering in the ruins of Hiroshima. In the end, he finds his young wife again but realises that he has lost his sexual potency.

This all throws a somewhat different light on the state of ecstatic pleasure that is sought in the mortal suffering that he inflicts on himself yet insists on sharing. Tanizaki's oeuvre caused a scandal in his lifetime because it illustrates all sorts of desires, often including the voluntary quest for exquisite pain by the victims who are always masters of their own martyrdom.

Masochism is enigmatic, and its very existence raises a question for psychoanalysis that Freud considered to be vital: *if pleasure and unpleasure are indistinguishable and coincide, what becomes, then, of the pleasure principle?*

Herein lies the economic problem of masochism, and the key text of 1924 could only envisage it by displacing the question of the strange relationship between pleasure and pain onto a radical re-examination of the entire psychoanalytic theory outlined hitherto.

It may, indeed, seem inconceivable that Freud – who was working on the theme of sexuality, which, as he had said in the *Three Essays on the Theory of Sexuality* (Freud, 1905) includes masochism – only discovered in

---

* This chapter was first published in 2000 under the title "L'énigme de la douleur" in J. André, editor, *L'énigme du masochisme*, Paris, Presses Universitaires de France.

DOI: 10.4324/9781003197652-2

1924 that defining the pleasure principle from the economic point of view alone makes masochism unintelligible.

Put more simply, it is surprising that pleasure, hitherto strictly equated with discharge, was opposed to unpleasure in the form of tension, retention and excitation; consequently, the fact that *there is pleasure in the tension of excitation* had been denied.

A retrospective reading of *Instincts and their Vicissitudes* (Freud, 1915) clearly shows that, before 1920, nothing was able to throw light on masochism as a clinical fact. It was not until the conception of something *Beyond the Pleasure Principle* (Freud, 1920) that the problem of masochism was finally posed heuristically.

The word *enigma* comes from αἴνιγμα in Greek, which implies, first of all, the idea of a detour. The meanings "obscure" and "mysterious" are a later semantic shift. With regard to the enigma in question, the necessary detour involved a revision of the first drive theory, which made it possible to think about self-destructiveness. The second drive opposition reunites, in the form of libido, the sexual drives and the self-preservative drives against the death drive – a force of unbinding, as defined by Freud (1940) in *An Outline of Psychoanalysis*.

This second drive theory brought in its wake the conception of the second topography, which is richer and more complex than the first, but above all raises certain issues differently. If the pleasure principle – hitherto considered as the guardian of psychic life – is indistinguishable from unpleasure, then unpleasure can become the aim of life. And Freud asked himself what the guardian of our psychic life would be. The answer lay in the twelve pages of the article of 1924 and involved the recognition of a primary erotogenic masochism that had hitherto been rejected. Henceforth, it was erotogenic masochism that became the guardian and guarantor of psychic life because it was the witness and vestigial trace of the alloy between the two instinctual drives: the libido, on the one hand, and the death drive, on the other. The fundamental notion of "drive fusion" had its origins here.

If the opposition between *sexuality* and *preservation* is replaced by the instinctual drive coupling of the *libido and* the *death drive*, we need to think, on the one hand, of libido in terms of frenzied binding, which, in order to avoid collusion and allow for desire, is opposed by a principle of unbinding that permits the long path of waiting. Yet the latter is unthinkable if we are unable to imagine a masochistic cathexis of unpleasure, a masochistic dimension of existence which makes the cathexis of the hallucination of pleasure possible.

Why do we not kill ourselves when faced with the first serious disappointment? Why do we enjoy suffering from love? Why? Because the fusion of the two antagonistic drives takes place on the basis of, and in accordance with, a primary erotogenic masochism which underpins the other forms of masochism: feminine, moral and secondary. The last of these is the turning round of sadism upon the subject's own self, which Freud described in 1915 as the sole form of *masochism*.

Readers who may want to study the different forms of masochism and its enigmas could usefully refer to two very different authors. One is Gilles Deleuze (1967), who shows that masochism is neither the antonym nor the complement of sadism, and that the entity "sadomasochism", invented by Krafft-Ebing, raises complex problems. There is no turning round but rather a double-paradoxical production. The sadistic partner of the masochist is an integral part of the masochistic scenario, and he has been educated to that end; he accepts the rules and cannot be thought of simply as a sadistic pervert. I do not agree with all the aspects of the critique that Deleuze makes of Freud's texts, but he nonetheless raises real questions.

The other is Benno Rosenberg (2003), with his remarkable monograph, as with his earlier articles. His central thesis is based on the hypothesis of a primal masochism binding destructiveness, which, once it is projected, becomes sadism. This conception makes it possible, in my opinion, to avoid the stumbling block of a genetic point of view such as Melanie Klein's. It also sees primary projection as the foundation of the later mechanisms of negation. Introjected sadism becomes auto-sadism, which, in turn, engenders guilt. The differentiation between moral masochism and the sense of guilt is thus announced in the dynamics between the ego and the superego. Masochism is a guardian of life not only because it primarily binds destructiveness; secondarily, it can also constitute an "attempt at healing". This explains the beginnings of perverse masochism in cold psychosis where self-destructive, self-mutilating behaviours could, due to their very excess, be seen as mitigating the deficiency of the initial masochistic nucleus.

Such an original theory of the constitution of the mind, based on a primal masochistic nucleus that organises hallucinatory wish-fulfilment and temporality, cannot fail to throw light on the two instinctual drive deviations in the form of somatosis and perverse acting out. Should we conclude that these two paths, or solutions, represent a challenge to what Rosenberg called the "masochistic dimension of existence"?

It is by recognising this "masochistic dimension" clinically that the validity of the concept of the death drive can again be justified: the primary ego is created from the initial narcissism, thanks to a "turning away" of a part of the death drive in order to serve the libido against attacks by the death drive. It is a matter of using the very essence of the death drive and its specificity by fundamentally reversing its aims. This "turning away" thus has an existential value and serves to ground negation.

I am in total agreement with Rosenberg with regard to the necessity of thinking through this masochistic dimension of existence, as well as that of the death drive. What is the source of the extraordinary robustness of the human mind which drives us to resist the worst calamities, both those that we produce ourselves and those caused by others, as well as sadism? How can we imagine life without suffering? How can we tolerate suffering if it is not intrinsically linked to the libido, and therefore eroticised?

The theory of the Paris Psychosomatic School, to which I adhere, as well as my clinical experience of extreme cases with patients suffering from painful, incapacitating or even deadly somatic illnesses, have led me to put forward the hypothesis of a *failure* of masochism, an existential dimension of the mind, and of masochism as a guardian of life, based on a failure of primary erotogenic masochism.

If the most eminent psychosomaticians of the first generation – in particular, Pierre Marty – did not often speak about masochism, it was because, when describing a new clinical field that is defined by a semiological void, narcissism and masochism are only expressed negatively. In fact, as early as "Narcissism: an introduction", Freud (1914) had referred to somatic illness and described the narcissistic backward flow that is necessary for fostering processes of healing. The withdrawal of narcissistic libido and the masochistic cathexis of the suffering body are indistinguishable here, but they are often absent in the somatic patients referred to by psychoanalysts, because in general they are the ones who cannot be helped adequately by classical medical therapeutic measures.

In these somewhat uncommon clinical pictures for psychoanalysts, anxiety and pain, too, are sometimes missing: are they anti-cathected, denied and anaesthetised? Yet masochism is the eroticised cathexis of suffering of which physical pain is the paradigm, since it refers to the model of the body.

Pain and the pleasure principle

Pain, as such, is difficult to think about and has not been explored much in psychoanalytic theory. There was entire volume of the *Revue française de psychosomatique* in 1999 that tackled the subject.[1] It seems to me, however, that a displacement of the "enigma of masochism" onto an "enigma of pain" can be found in Freud's work and after the turning-point of 1920.

From the moment Freud accepted that masochism – a clinical fact – thwarted his strictly economic conception of the pleasure principle, he revised it by *rehabilitating excitation*. The tension of excitation, albeit painful, contains pleasure. This leads on to the subversive idea that the masochistic pleasure of pain became (after "The economic problem of masochism" and in the second drive theory) the very model of pleasure. Curiously enough, in the *Three Essays . . .*, Freud (1905) was close to this way of seeing things, but subsequently abandoned it. It seems to me that, in so doing, he dropped the term *"enigmatic"* and accepted the paradox of masochism as such. What remained enigmatic was pain in itself, which is always marked by the two poles of pleasure and that which is beyond it.

I am thus taking the risk here of speaking about pain, about its clinical features, and even its theory, as models and substrata of all forms of suffering.

In attempting to approach the essence of it, I will draw on three sources: a literary text, a film (and the article devoted to it by a psychoanalyst) and, lastly, certain clinical cases of somatic patients.

It is worth recalling here that Freud, who was himself a specialist of psychic and moral pain, began his career by studying an anaesthetic substance: cocaine. The anaesthesia that Freud refers to in Draft G constitutes a protection against the unbearable aspects of the drive, "but everything that encourages anaesthesia provokes the development of melancholia" (see Masson, 1985, p. 98), he wrote to Fliess, thereby emphasising the paradox linked from the outset to pain, even if to its negative: anaesthesia (Lubstchansky, 1999).

On this theme, precisely, Nikolaj Frobenius, a Norwegian novelist, portrays in a striking manner the development of a child born in Honfleur in the 18th century with a defect: he feels no pain. The author tells us about the unhappiness of this child, named Latour:

> What is pain?
>
> Latour thought there were four different types of pain. Everyday pain. Deep-rooted pain. The pain that came from heart and stomach. And the pain that came from thinking too much. He never ceased to be amazed at the grimaces on Bou-Bou's face whenever she had sore blisters. He felt nothing himself, and sometimes wondered if he was fully alive. . . . The mental pain that Latour had felt when Goupils tied him to the tree in the garden and made him wait there for a punishment that never materialized was for him a false and unpleasant pain. It was impossible to control and made him wish he were dead. . . . He also felt another kind of mental pain . . . this was the pain you feel when you know you are enslaved by something you do not understand.
>
> (Frobenius, 2000, p. 40)

Obsessed by what he experiences as an infirmity, the young Latour tortures insects, dissects and kills them. He wants to understand something about human nature that eludes him constantly. He develops an obsession for anatomy, becomes the assistant of the famous and controversial anatomist Rochefoucault, and finally meets the Marquis de Sade, who makes him his valet.

Nikolaj Frobenius offers us a romantic and period fresco, but also shows the implacable internal compulsion that leads Latour to sadism in a tragic destiny, insofar as all pleasure or play are absent from it.

I would like to contrast this suffering linked to the absence of pain with another conception of pain as "therapeutics of survival". Patrick Miller (1999), the author of this expression, comments on an almost unbearable 1997 film, *Sick: The Life and Death of Bob Flanagan: Supermasochist*, directed by Kirby Dick, in which Bob Flanagan is the main protagonist. He suffers from cystic fibrosis, a lethal disease to which those who suffer from it usually succumb before the age of twenty-five. Bob Flanegan was 43 years old when he participated in this film, aimed at showing how he kept himself alive by making his body an object of torture, like a work of art.

This same theme combining sadomasochism, sublimation and death is also the theme of a very fine short story by Jun'ichirō Tanizaki (1914), "A Golden Death", in which the hero subjects himself to a slow and painful death during a glorious spectacle. The difference with the film about Flanegan lies in the latter's relentless struggle against a foretold death through the enactment of a perverse scenario which involved approaching death – via the pain inflicted – through pleasure and desire. Notwithstanding the unbearable images, it is more of a tragic testimony than a perverse film that puts the spectator in the position of a voyeur. The article devoted by Miller to it shows with great subtlety how the encounter with Flanagan's sadomasochistic partner is crucial, and how this woman seeks desperately to keep him alive by keeping the game going, reviving the masochistic mode of functioning relentlessly. Miller suggests that pain acts here as a drive; that is, as a pseudo-drive. This is in keeping with Freudian theory of a countercharge, elaborated to account for what is beyond the pleasure principle. The irruption of stimuli provoked by the biological defect must be countered by introducing eroticised physical pain.

Less extreme is the last example, a clinical case of an analysand, whom I have called Taëko, after the heroine of the 1963 novel by Yukio Mishima (1993), called *L'École de la chair* [The School of Flesh], the title of which sums up quite well the path that disease, and then analysis, made this woman follow.

The school of flesh

The "school of flesh", for her, involved experiencing disease. In the case of this woman, it is on the sick body that an erotic body (Fain & Dejours, 1984) is built. This, at least, is my hypothesis today.

Taëko was diagnosed with cervical cancer a little before the age of thirty-six. The prognosis for this form of cancer is generally very favourable; however, the doctors had been worried by the patient's age and the fact that she had reached stage 4 from a histological point of view. Her husband, a biology researcher, recommended that she have a hysterectomy, while the first gynaecologist she had seen had advised her to have the cervix removed completely. The second had suggested having a wide conisation of the cervix followed by radiotherapy. Taëko told me she had fought to keep a part of her cervix. She had astonished herself. Due to her youth, the radiotherapy was replaced by chemotherapy, which she said was "horrific", leaving her with so much pain and feeling very nauseous. She had experienced this whole period as a serious threat to her sexual life and to her life, full stop. She thought she only had three or four years of life left and that she had to live them intensely. It was during this same period that she decided to get divorced. She had been married for fifteen years to a man sixteen years older than her. He was the first man she had known, and she had loved him.

Taëko did not have any children and mentioned with a certain lightness and without dwelling on them two miscarriages. She told me about a psychoanalytic psychotherapy that she had done for two years and which had helped her a great deal between the ages of eighteen and twenty. She had sought help with intellectual inhibitions, difficulty in working and a general sense of being ill-at-ease in her body. She had been clumsy, awkward and ungraceful. During puberty, she had become overweight; ever since, Taëko had felt she was ugly and stupid. She dreamed of being rid of this heavy body that hindered her capacity to think.

She recalled her first meeting with the analyst, who was an elderly man. She had said to him: "I hate my body and I loathe my father". He had smiled, apparently. The psychotherapy was miraculous: she left "cured", passed all her exams and got married shortly after.

I asked Taëko if she had been happy in her marriage. A little surprised, she replied that, at the time, she had not asked herself this question. Everything had gone well and things seemed to be in place "for eternity". The news of the cancer, which had come like a clap of thunder, a menace from the outside, had upset this fixed, and therefore precarious, equilibrium. Taëko lived outside time, but now the notion of a "time limit" had been imposed on her suddenly. She noted that she had been astonished at the time to see how women were terrified of ageing. Being "ageless", she did not think she would be affected by it. I linked this remark to the two miscarriages, pointing out to her that being a mother herself implied entering the succession of generations and time. The reason for seeking treatment was not in order to understand why she had developed cancer at the age of thirty-six, after two spontaneous terminations of pregnancies, for which no medical causes had been diagnosed. Taëko was suffering from anxiety – diffuse and constant anxiety that plunged her into a strange state of mind. But this was now that she was cured and free because she was divorced, still young and without children. "Anything can happen", I said to her, "unlike in eternity".

Very quickly, in the second preliminary interview, Taëko became aware that she was plagued by both violent and vague sexual desires. We agreed on her doing an analysis. I recall telling myself that she needed to be able to cry. Her "Japanese" self-containment, which I thought was probably equal to the underlying violence, suggested to me that she could not work face-to-face. It seemed to me that Taëko, at this moment in her life, was not so much a clear indication for a classical analysis as a counter-indication for psychotherapy, since there was a danger that an improvement of her symptoms would leave her, once again, fixed in an unstable equilibrium. It was necessary, in my view, to take into account a deep process that her illness had already set in process. Taëko had thought she was invulnerable, and for a long time, had denied the castration of ageing. She had previously never been able to get in touch with her depressive tendencies, but the illness, the chemotherapy, the painful attack on her body, the loss of her hair, had obliged her to do so. I therefore made the informed but perhaps more risky choice of doing a classical analysis.

In the early stages, she talked a lot about her divorce. She spoke of it as a violent but necessary separation. Her husband had failed her in her illness. No doubt in a state of panic, he either dramatised the situation – "A complete hysterectomy so as to on the safe side." – or was in denial about it – "It's nothing, just a small setback". He decided to leave for Harvard for three months in the context of an exchange between teachers and researchers. His wife's support prevented him from even imagining showing her his disappointment, but he began to withdraw emotionally from her. This behaviour reminded Taëko of her own mother, who had often been absent, without Taëko being aware of the reasons for her travels. Her mother, who was sweet and discreet, would constantly go away, leaving an imposing father entirely free to pamper this youngest daughter, who was born later, after three boys. He would choose her dresses, take her to the theatre or to dine in top restaurants. She would have liked her to have a literary bent so that she could collaborate with him in his publishing house.

Owing to the difference in age between them, Taëko thought she had probably been looking for a father in her husband. However, like her mother, he was one of these enigmatic individuals who withdraw from the relationship if it is not confined within strict boundaries. She said she knew nothing about him. When she was thirty-five, she described a certain tension that had come between them when they found themselves alone. I tried to understand why this had occurred, precisely, in that year. A story she recounted in snippets, and initially without affects, gave meaning to the sequence of cancer-divorce. The only daughter of four children, Taëko had formed an affectionate and tender friendship with Mathilde, her sister-in-law. This sister of her husband was the youngest child; there were ten years between her and her elder brother. She was therefore six years older than Taëko. Sharing close professional interests, the two sisters-in-law had become inseparable; they travelled together, laughed a lot and disappeared on Sundays to see three films in a row, like adolescents.

Two years earlier – Taëko was therefore thirty-four – Mathilde had met a man and, although their relationship had been stormy, she had left everything to follow him abroad. Taëko was dumfounded by this "madness". Five years later, in the analysis, it took her time to get in touch with the feelings of rage, rancour and homosexual disappointment that she had suppressed. At the time, she had apparently withdrawn her interest in Mathilde, but finding herself face-to-face with her husband had become difficult. Aside from the sorrow of a sentimental order, she had lost an identificatory support from someone who was warmer than her mother, because there had been a feminine intimacy between Mathilde and Taëko. It was in this connection that I learnt that, as a young girl, Taëko had fled from women. Her friendships, all cerebral moreover, had all been with men. She had experienced the onset of her first menstrual periods as shameful, compounded by a sense of injustice: "Why me, and not my brothers?" The psychotherapy, when she was eighteen, had helped her to understand that trying to protect herself by putting on weight was useless, and that thinking and learning would not necessarily land her in her father's arms. She had then found a man whom she thought was invulnerable because he was distant, and an equilibrium between this man and Mathilde that was too stable: time had no place in it. Her unconscious refusal to have a child was interpreted along these lines.

Taëko's anxiety abated early on in the analysis when she became aware of her desires and a formidable appetite for living. Since her illness, she felt she had a body – a woman's body – and pictured it to herself. The cancer had given her a belly, a uterus and a cervix, she said. She liked her hair that she had lost and recovered. Sometimes, she seemed to me to be in a state of joyful overexcitement; I could not help wondering if it was defensive, and feared above all that it might lead to the onset of a depression as a "cover" (Aisenstein, 1988) for ceasing to desire.

In the analysis, there had been little mention so far of her parents during her childhood. The material was lively, interesting and associative, and yet the infantile neurosis and the organisation of mental life by primal fantasies seemed to be missing. One day, when she was sobbing in connection with a dream she had had in which Mathilde did not recognise her in the street, I said to her: "And yet she is not the first woman in your life". Taëko broke down; she had not known her mother, who had never recognised her. She hated her. The classical interpretation in the transference would have been that I might not greet her in the street as one normally would greet an acquaintance. However, such an intervention seemed to me to be premature. So, I chose a formulation that was more in the order of a reconstruction.

During this period, she also had several dreams that she called "anxiety dreams", but in fact they were typical dreams of nudity. She saw herself half-naked; she had forgotten either her dress or her blouse and so felt frightened and shameful. One night, she had a nightmare: her husband was holding a brunette in his arms. She awoke with a start in a state of jealousy, and her heart was beating wildly. In the meantime, she had come cross an old friend from the past again, called René; they had shared the same literary interests. He was married and fully occupied with caring for his wife, who was suffering from advanced multiple sclerosis. Taëko and this man began a discreet and passionate relationship, which satisfied her completely. Gradually and firmly, but not abruptly, this man introduced Taëko to other women; never the same ones, all younger and often exotic. They were transient women, sometimes professional prostitutes and sometimes women he had had an indulgent adventure with the evening before. Through this sexuality, where she submitted to all her lover's desires, Taëko said that she had attained heights of pleasure she had not known before, but suffered at the same time from pangs of jealousy, a feeling that was totally new for her, except in her dreams. She was tortured for nights on end by the idea that René might be seeing one of these women without her. Finally, she recalled that, once in her childhood, she had screamed alone in the dark on hearing laughter coming from her parents' bedroom.

The feelings that she shared with her lover went beyond those of a perverse relationship, and she obtained protection and tenderness from him until the day he broke off the relationship. He suggested that they continued to be friends, but she declined. The reason he gave for terminating the relationship was a sudden deterioration in his wife's condition. He said he did not want to share the last moments of her life with anyone else. All this made Taëko feel "ill" – it was her word – ill with despair, jealousy, envy towards this woman who was dying, but who was a *mother* and dependent on a man. She imagined scenarios in which she was going to kill them, shoot them both at point blank range, have poisoned meals delivered to them and so on. She cried a lot.

"This is making me ill", she said.
"But from love this time", I pointed out to her.
"It's the same thing. Without the cancer, I wouldn't have had a belly
   and I wouldn't have had René", she replied impulsively.

The loss of a living man obliged her to go through a real process of mourning; her de-cathected state was over. It was once again her body that alerted her to the end of her depression. "I woke up with a frenetic desire to go running in the country. If I have such desires, it means that I am no longer ill. I can get by without René by myself".

In the final session, the last dream of the analysis did not need commenting on: she felt heavy and ponderous, but strangely enough, it was quite a pleasant feeling. She went and stood in front of a mirror and she thought she looked pregnant, but she was filled with a feeling of plenitude. She saw me arriving in the mirror. I was the one who said goodbye because I had an appointment. Taëko said, "Pregnant with the child that I will not have; but nevertheless, I have lots of things in my belly and now, I know both how to lose and to keep. It took all this time".

I noted the appearance of a reflection of herself in the mirror in a dream, as well as the theme of time, the denial of which had, in my view, masked a denial of castration.

Some questions

Although a strict setting was respected, this analysis did not seem so classical to me. Event-related material played a great role in it; however, this is not equivalent to the factual and raises the question of the libidinal sympathetic excitation and somatic excitation that are indispensable to the drive. This brings us back to the theme of illness.

Even when it arises from a disorganisation, somatic illness can – in my view – induce from the outside, as it were, a masochistic re-sexualisation and possibilities of regression. Disorganisations can become regressions during the analysis. Furthermore, I think that illness can become a factor of psychic reorganisation independently of analysis. Retrospectively, the event is reintegrated within an elaborative psychic chain. If it is not disorganising – and that is a question of quantity – pain becomes suffering, and thus, a demand for representation. This representation forces masochistic cathexis. In other words, should we not ask ourselves if the excess itself, the masochistic profusion of pain that a serious illness can make the patient go through, does not constitute an attempt to heal the initial failure of the primary masochistic nucleus as an organiser? It seems to me that, through the attack of illness and lack, the integration of a narcissism that is initially defensive with a masochism as the guardian of life is conceivable.

At a strictly economic level, can somatosis not be seen as binding this "indifferent, displaceable energy" described by Freud (1923) in *The Ego and the Id*? (p. 44)? In this text, Freud discusses how the excesses of external and internal stimuli turn parts of the ego into parts of the id. The fate of a force liberated in this way can follow various paths. After her illness, when she felt pulled in all directions by her desires, Taëko chose the long path of psychic elaboration in analysis rather than of exhaustion through discharge. She had sought analysis on account of diffuse anxieties, but during it she had become acquainted with pain and lack.

"Anxiety, pain and mourning" is the title given by Freud (1926) to the Addenda C that concludes *Inhibitions, Symptoms and Anxiety*. Bodily pain causes a narcissistic cathexis of the painful zone. When internal organs, which are ordinarily not represented, are the source of pain, they are the object of "spatial and other presentations". On the other hand, even the most intense physical pains are sometimes not felt if the mind is distracted at that moment by other interests. This is accounted for by there being a concentration of cathexis on the psychical representative of the part of the body that is painful. And Freud concludes:

> I think it is here that we shall find the point of analogy which has made it possible to carry sensations of pain over to the mental sphere. For the intense cathexis of longing which is concentrated on the missed or lost object (a cathexis which readily mounts up because it cannot be appeased) creates the same economic conditions as are created by the cathexis of pain which is concentrated on the injured part of the body. . . . The transition from physical pain to mental pain corresponds to a change from narcissistic cathexis to object-cathexis.
>
> (Freud, 1926, p. 171)

In a passage in Book II of the *Tusculan Disputations*, at the beginning of section XV "On bearing pain", Cicero (1877, p. 78) criticises the Stoics:

"Both these feelings [labour and pain], the Greeks, whose language is more copious than ours, express by the common name Πόνος". He is surprised by this semantic condensation, which he regards as one of the paradoxes of Greek thought.

Although research in psychoanalysis often faces us with enigma and paradox, the idea that thought is both painful and extremely pleasurable comes as no surprise for psychoanalysts.

Note

1 "Douleurs", *Revue française psychosomatique*, 15, Autumn 1999.

References

Aisenstein, M. (1988). Une histoire de rouge à lèvres. *Les Cahiers du Centre de psychanalyse* 16–17: 87–106.

Cicero, M. T. (1877). *Tusculan Disputations*, trans. C. D. Yonge. New York, NY: Harper Brothers.

Deleuze, G. (1967). *Présentation de Sacher-Masoch*. Paris: Minuit.

Fain, M., & Dejours, C. (1984). *Corps malade et corps érotique*. Paris: Masson.

Freud, S. (1905). *Three Essays on the Theory of Sexuality*. S.E., 7. London: Hogarth, pp. 123–243.

Freud, S. (1914). *Narcissism: An Introduction*. S.E., 14. London: Hogarth, pp. 69–102.

Freud, S. (1915). *Instincts and their Vicissitudes*. S.E., 14. London: Hogarth, pp. 109–140.

Freud, S. (1920). *Beyond the Pleasure Principle*. S.E., 18. London: Hogarth, pp. 1–64.

Freud, S. (1923). *The Ego and the Id*. S.E., 19. London: Hogarth, pp. 3–66.

Freud, S. (1926). *Inhibitions, Symptoms and Anxiety*. S.E., 20. London: Hogarth, pp. 75–174.

Freud, S. (1940). *An Outline of Psychoanalysis*. S.E., 23. London: Hogarth, pp. 139–207.

Frobenius, N. (2000/1996). *Sade's Valet*. London: Blackwell.

Lubstchansky, J. (1999). Insoutenable immaturité de l'être. *Revue française de psychosomatique* 1(15): 175–194.

Masson, J. M. (Ed.). (1985). *The Complete Letters of Sigmund Freud to Wilhelm Fliess, 1887–1904*. Cambridge, MA: Belknap.

Miller, P. (1999). La douleur: une thérapeutique de survie? Quelques éléments de réflexion. *Revue française de psychosomatique* 15: 39–50.

Mishima, Y. (1993/1963). *L'École de la chair*. Paris: Gallimard.

Rosenberg, B. (2003). Masochisme mortifère, masochisme gardien de vie. In: *Monograph of the Revue française de psychanalyse*, B. Rosenberg. Paris: Presses Universitaires Françaises, pp. 55–91.

Tanizaki, J. (1914/2013). Une mort dorée. In: *Le secret et autres textes*, ed. J. Tanizaki. Paris: Gallimard, pp. 1616–1638.

Tanizaki, J. (1997–1998). *Chroniques inhumaines, 1943–1951, Œuvres*, Vol. 2. Paris: Gallimard, La Pléiade, pp. 1125–1191.

2   The birth of desire

The word "desire" makes me think irresistibly of "love". This is why, before looking at the Freudian theory of desire, I would like to say a few words about the love letters that the young Freud and his fiancée Martha wrote to each other during the four years of their engagement between 1882 and 1886. There are 1,500 letters in all, which are in the Library of Congress in Washington, D.C. Ilse Grubrich-Simitis who, in 2003, gave a remarkable lecture in Mexico on this correspondence, is working on its publication and has already published the first of five volumes in German under the title "Be mine in the way I imagine it" (Grubrich-Simitis et al., 2011). Clearly, desire is very much present in love, along with dreaming and thinking. The theories of wishful hallucination and of representation (of words and things) are already present in embryonic form in the exchanges between the two lovers. I will just give a limited sample of them here.

In June 1884, Martha wrote, "I already welcome you in my dreams every night. So, isn't it strange that during the last few days I was absolutely convinced that you would not come?" Shortly after, telling her about his visit to the Notre Dame tower in Paris, Freud said, "On each step, I could have given you a kiss, if you had been there, and you would have arrived at the top completely out of breath and wild" (ibid.).

Need and desire: Freudian theory

I am going to try to summarise in simple words the schema of desire in Freud's work. To do this, I will refer to two fundamental texts: the "Project for a scientific psychology" (1950 [1895]) and Chapter VII of *The Interpretation of Dreams* (1900). Then I will give a personal reading of the notion of "hallucinatory wish-fulfilment", which will lead me to elaborate briefly on a later text, "The economic problem of masochism" (1924).

As early as 1895, in the "Project", Freud elaborated a theory of desire beginning with the early stages of the human organism. The helpless infant is subjected to distressing stimuli; for example, hunger, which can only be alleviated by a specific external action: breastfeeding. In the infant, a *memory image* is created, which associates this experience of satisfaction

DOI: 10.4324/9781003197652-3

with the desired object. These experiences leave traces which are *affects of unpleasure* and *states of wishing* (*états de désir*). These are characterised by an increase of internal tension, followed by a sudden liberation. To put it differently, an experience of "craving" creates tension in the ego which is subsequently associated with the cathexis of the desired object. For the infant, it is at first milk and the mother, who gives him the breast. This cathexis is what we call a "wishful idea" (*représentation de désir*).

Whilst initially this schema seems very simple, it becomes increasingly more complex. How does the transition from the milk to the mother as an object of desire, and then to the representation of the mother, occur? First, it is important to differentiate between *need* and *desire*. Need is vital and corresponds to a necessity that implies its biological root: if deprived of food, a baby will die. Desire, on the other hand, is a powerful and sometimes violent feeling that attests to the strength of the drive. It is psychic work that allows for the transition from need to desire. In order for this transition to take place, distressing stimuli must be calmed by an "experience of satisfaction" that has been memorised. This memorisation will then arouse an attraction towards the object, and it is this movement towards the object that we call "desire". Desire is born of need. Next, the recognition of desire will give rise to the recognition of the object and, consequently, the birth of the desiring subject.

As I mentioned earlier, the Freudian conception of "hallucinatory wish-fulfilment" becomes clearer on reading the "The psychology of the dream-processes", Chapter VII of *The Interpretation of Dreams*, where Freud (1900) returns to the schema described in the "Project", backing it up by the clinical experience of dreams. The latter has the advantage, moreover, of integrating both conscious desire and unconscious wishes. The dream is a "wish-fulfilment": he presents the facts as the dreamer would have liked them to have unfolded.

I will not dwell further here on this famous Chapter VII. On the other hand, I would like to insist on the dream as a model of "hallucinatory wish-fulfilment", because it is at the foundation of fantasy life and thought, which are specific characteristics of the human being and therefore of the desiring subject.

Let us return to the example of the baby who is hungry. Hunger is a need which, thanks to the registration of the memory-trace of satisfaction, is transformed into desire. There is a first transition from the *need for milk* to the desire for the breast; then, a second transition from *expectation of the breast* to that of the object-mother: these transitions imply psychic work. As in dreams, but in the waking state, the hungry infant hallucinates and imagines his mother arriving. The desiring infant thereby gains access to thought.

Freud (1900) writes, "Thought is after all nothing but a substitute for a hallucinatory wish; and it is self-evident that dreams must be wish-fulfilments, since nothing but a wish can set our mental apparatus at work"

(p. 567). This statement is crucial because it implies and emphasises the fact that desire is the ground of psychic work and thought. However, there is one point that seems to me to be obscure in Freud's text, even though I must have read it hundreds of times: how does the transition from urgent need to desire – that is to say, to the capacity for thinking and waiting – occur in the infant? Personally, it is once again in the light of the text of 1924, and in particular of the notion of "primary erotogenic masochism", that I manage to understand the birth of desire in the mind of the child.

For Freud, this primary masochism is very early, and it makes it possible to bind contradictory drive impulses in the child's ego. To put it simply, by binding the libido (a force that pushes) and the death drive (a movement that unbinds and immobilises), primary masochism makes it possible to integrate the capacity for waiting. This obviously comes about by virtue of the mother's psychic work. A "good enough mother" is one who, through her words, can induce the child to wait: "Wait my little one; I'm going to take you in my arms, but not immediately. I will give you the bottle soon, stay calm, wait a little". The mother envelops the child with words, she gives him word- and thing-presentations and thus helps him to wait, which implies trust in the object.

Why is the concept of primary masochism indispensable here? Because waiting must be "masochistically cathected" if it is to become tolerable. The infant must gradually understand that *there is also pleasure* in waiting, *precisely because of the psychic work that it implies*. This *cathexis of delay* is what grounds desire: I think about and imagine the pleasure to come.

I say quite readily that the "structure of desire is masochistic in essence", because it is not conceivable without renouncing immediateness and without cathecting waiting. The lover who will see the object of his desire in one week, or in a month, is able to tolerate waiting because he has learnt to find pleasure in psychic work and in his fantasy scenarios of the meeting to come. This is what Freud did when he wrote to Martha: "One day you will be mine in the way I imagine it".

From non-desire to the recognition of desire

In classical patients (more or less neurotic organisations), desire and psychic work exist from the outset in analysis. The transference is based on desire. But many so-called "difficult" patients (borderline, psychosomatic or "operational" (*opératoire*)) organise their psychic life "against desire". They defend themselves in this way against the object.

I have chosen to present here a fragment of a treatment of a patient who drove me to despair because she was and claimed to be "without love and without desire". She had been referred to me by her doctors, who were worried about her somatic fragility.

A beating heart

When she was thirty-two, she had suffered from breast cancer. Then, during the eighteen months that followed her treatment, involving a mastectomy and chemotherapy, she had had two strokes.

Carla was a young, sportive-looking, fair-haired woman; she was thirty-four when she began face-to-face psychoanalytic therapy with me. She told me that she had come to see me because she trusted her doctors, but she could not believe in psychoanalysis; she felt she had no problems, anxieties or depression. She said she did not like to dwell on herself too much: "I don't like thinking and prefer action". In fact, she was a professional sportswoman and had no social or erotic life. She did not try to make friends because she soon felt invaded by the presence of other people. Her very ascetic life revolved around her training sessions, which exhausted her, though she had no complaints about that.

In view of her fear of being intruded upon, I suggested we begin with just one session per week. Carla accepted and did not show any signs of scepticism, reticence or mistrust. For a long time, her discourse was very factual, without affect and "operational" in style; but she seemed to enjoy coming, did not miss any sessions, and even asked for a second session of her own accord. At the end of the first year, she was surprised to be having so many dreams.

Her first dream was of a *snowy, white landscape; everything was still and icy, but the snow was not cold.* I pointed out to her that there was no one in the dream. "Yes, it's like a still life", she replied. I suggested that this dream could be understood as a picture of her emotional life: immobile and iced up. I added, "But it doesn't seem to be either cold or hot". The patient was moved and said, "You know, when I was about twelve years old, I 'lost the hot and the cold'". As I was surprised by this unusual formulation, she explained that, shortly after her first periods, she stopped having a sense of temperatures; she didn't feel the sensation of boiling water, didn't feel the cold in winter, and so on. "It was like that".

I suggested that it was as if she had been *anaesthetised*. In the following sessions, I learnt that, before "the loss of the hot and the cold", her father had died accidentally. Now she began to recall her childhood. Her mother had been a hard and violent woman who used to "scream and hit her the whole time" (five years later I learned that the mother had virtually become a nymphomaniac, receiving a variety of lovers while her daughter was locked up in the kitchen).

Carla had not forgotten anything, but she never thought about it. It was all "frozen, anaesthetised". It was not repression that was involved, but rather a drastic suppression aimed at warding off affect, which explained the "struggle against thinking", her tendency to discharge her feelings in action and all the exhausting physical exercise. From a psychosomatic point of view, the sequence that I have described as "somatic disorganisation" (cancer and two strokes) had followed a bad fracture that had immobilised her and stopped her from doing any sport for more than six months, thereby barring all her usual paths of discharge.

A second period of analytic work also began with a dream. It was after my summer holiday, in the third year of treatment. She was having sessions three times a week, face-to-face. At the beginning of the session, she told me the following dream: *I dreamt that I was falling asleep; I was fighting against invasive and dangerous feelings of drowsiness; I succumbed, and a black veil was going to cover my head. I was afraid and felt that my brain was caught in a net; it was going to be numb forever. Was it my stroke? Was it death? I struggled to wake up during the dream. Then I woke up for real. I was all clammy and my heart was beating fast; I turned the light on, went to the bathroom, and then drank some water. Strangely, that calmed me down.*

I said, "Because you could see that you were still alive, physically and mentally".

"Ah, I have forgotten a bit of the dream", she replied. "I managed to wake up, perhaps because a man I didn't know came into the room and held out his hand to me; it was reassuring".

I thought to myself: a man she doesn't know, the opposite of a woman she knows, but who is absent because she's on holiday. I was caught up in a network of associations: her strokes and the fear that they aroused in me, and the constant state of alert I was in with this patient. The black veil, the title of a novel (*Le voile noir*) by Annie Dupérey[1] (1992), also reminded me of a very old Greek film in which Clytemnestra had Agamemnon entangled in a big cloth net while he was asleep in his bath so that she could kill him. I thought about the patient's first dream (the still life), which had seemed to me to depict her mental functioning. I was struck by the idea: "It's a soul murder".

After I had reminded her that she was alive, she recalled the fragment, "a man I didn't know came into the room and held out his hand to me; it was reassuring". In her short childhood nightmares, which always woke her up with a start, there was a disturbing, unknown man. This was why I was interested in the reversal: an unknown man and not a familiar woman. I found myself thinking again about the Greek film and the murderous expression of Clytemnestra, who ordered her lover, Aegisthus, to put the net over Agamemnon. In the whirlwind of my emotions, Clytemnestra seemed like my patient's mother. I told myself that I hated this woman and that I was afraid for my patient. I felt guilty for having gone away on holiday. And what if, instead of a dream, she had had another stroke? I thought about her father, who had died in an accident; he was absent and had left her to this soul-murdering mother. She told me so little about her father that I could not imagine his face. *The man in the dream reminded me that there was no man in her life or in her head.* I found this distressing. Did I have sexuality sufficiently in my mind with her? At this point, I noticed that Carla was crying silently. Tears were running down her face. She said,

"These strokes . . . the idea of having a scar in the brain. It hurt so much. Just six months after the end of the chemotherapy, it was too much. I don't like to think about it". She told me for the second time about her first stroke, but this time, her account was very different; it was full of affect.

While she was recovering from her breast cancer, she was woken up by a penetrating pain in her head: "It wasn't a headache, but an unimaginable pain". She wanted to get up but felt dizzy. She was taken to hospital. The diagnosis was always a bit vague, but the presence of a scar from recent bleeding was confirmed. "I don't know, I don't want to think about it", she said, "but it was worse than having two cancers".

I felt very weak, as if I was going to faint. I thought to myself that, although she often played down her illnesses, she must have in her an "experience of slipping away from life", of fainting (which she was communicating to me), closely linked to the "anaesthesia" of affects, but also to her experience of anaesthesia during her operations, repeated by the strokes.

I was in complete disarray and said to her, "A scar from bleeding in the brain makes me think of the blood of your first periods. It was just after that that you experienced an anaesthesia of hot and cold sensations, and you are so afraid of the sleep-induced anaesthesia". Carla understood very well; she sobbed and said to me, "And I thought that there was nothing going on in my head".

I have related the session of the "black veil" to show where we were in the process, but the session I want to report in detail occurred roughly a year later, towards the beginning of the fifth year. I would like to use this session to illustrate clinically what I mean by "levels or strata" of the transference.

The patient was still being followed by two hospital medical teams of neurologists and cardiologists. She had been advised to see a specialist in cardiac arrhythmias, whom she did not know. She told me in a light-hearted tone that Professor R. had asked her if she had had paroxysmal tachycardia for a long time. She had replied, "Yes, since adolescence; how did you know that?"

Totally shocked and fuming with anger inwardly, I said to her, "Are you telling me that you've had paroxysmal tachycardia since adolescence and that you've been hiding it from me as well as from your doctors?"

"Yes", Carla replied, "but I wasn't able to put it into words for myself. At first, I didn't hide it, and then afterwards, I didn't want to share this thing".

I was shocked, in view of the serious health risk that she was running like this, and asked her to explain things more clearly. I understood that, when she had had her first bouts of tachycardia, she hadn't given it any thought. She had simply experienced them and "liked it". Later, when questioned by her doctors, she realised that she should have told them about it, but feared that they would be taken away from her.

Interested by her admission that she "liked it", I noticed that my own heart was beating faster, which I thought was probably linked to my anger. I felt that she had deceived me: she had hidden, even from me, the pleasure she had derived from a symptom that was reminiscent of the state of being in love. I put this to her by saying, "While, for months you've been telling me that there is no man or woman in your life who makes your heart throb, you have been enjoying paroxysmal heart beats all by yourself. You are in love without sharing it with anyone".

Dumbfounded, Carla looked at me, breaking into laughter, and said, "I would never have thought about it like that".

She seemed cheerful, and it was only after a very long silence that, taking up the material again, I completed my interpretation by suggesting that she had now recovered from her "anaesthesia" and was hiding her heartbeats from me because they were perhaps connected with me.

This session marked a turning-point in this fascinating treatment, which lasted eight years.

Desire and transference

Transference implies an object and a desiring subject. I mean that interpreting the transference is only possible here after it has been dissected.

She can feel things in her body, but has no words for them. Then she has the words and can transform "this thing" into word- and thing-presentations. It is only after the transposition into language that the space of polysemy (tachycardia/her heart beating with love) can open up; but the object to whom she can address these words is still lacking. Yet the displacement that defines the transference requires an object to make itself available.

A detour via unconscious perception

Very recently, when I was worried about one of my relatives, a psychotic female patient, who also suffers from insulin-dependent diabetes and severe asthma, said to me at the beginning of a session, "A great sense of sadness came over me as soon as I entered the room; it's to do with illness and death ... I can't think about anything else". As I remained silent, she began to talk about the long illness of her grandfather, whom she had never spoken about before. It seemed obvious to me that she had noticed something that concerned me and that this was inevitably going to orient the material. I think it is necessary to accept that this is the case but that it is better not to respond.

These phenomena concerning unconscious perception are at the heart of the countertransference and exist in every analysis. They are very discreet in classical analyses, where the process of putting things into words and ideational activity are favoured by associations, but they take on great importance in the technique of more "difficult" treatments. This is because the transference is not only "libidinal" but also "beyond the pleasure principle"; but, above all, because the conversion from the psychic apparatus on to language, containing infinite metaphorical possibilities, cannot be taken for granted.

I think that, with these borderline patients whose mental organisation is not characterised by an Oedipal solution that is a mark of neurotic and elaborative capacities, receptivity to the unconscious of the other, of the analyst – that is, of the cathected object – is increased. This enigma of the sensitivity of certain patients to the analyst's unconscious-preconscious system has been nagging me for a long time. Pierre Marty used to say in supervisions, "Be careful, their unconscious does not emit, but receives". How is this clinical phenomenon to be understood?

In his text "The unconscious", Freud (1915) explains that the preconscious protects itself against the pressure of ideas by an anti-cathexis fuelled precisely by the energy that is withdrawn from ideas. In the two short examples related above, we witness a sudden impulse to act out in one and a surge of anxiety in the other in connection with an affective state of the analyst: an unconscious perception in them of an affect in me. I would say that, with Carla, there is an unconscious circulation consisting of perceptions between the two of us. But if the repressed idea remains in the unconscious as a real formation, the unconscious affect is just a "rudiment" charged with energy which seeks to break through the barrier of the preconscious.

In Chapter VII of *The Interpretation of Dreams*, Freud (1900) studies "the communication between the two systems". Each transition from one system to another involves a change of cathexis. This does not suffice, however, to explain the constant nature of primal repression. It is therefore necessary to assume that there is a process that makes the latter endure. Here, Freud puts forward the idea that the preconscious protects itself from the pressure of ideas, thanks to an anti-cathexis which draws its energy from the source of ideas. It is my contention that, in certain patients, this anti-cathexis is so drastic that it paralyses the preconscious and isolates the unconscious. However, these same patients cathect the outside world, and they compulsively cathect the object – that is to say, the analyst. But here, in the first stage of intersubjective relations, this drastic anti-cathexis concerns the internal, endo-psychic world. On the other hand, it is without effect on what comes from the cathected external object. If this crucial notion of "unconscious perception" is accepted, it could explain the hypersensitivity of these patients and their acute perception of others.

Desire is masochistic in essence because it implies waiting, the putting into abeyance of all action and psychic work. Similarly, the transference, which is the only instrument of analysis, is only conceivable when the patient becomes a desiring subject.

Note

1 A well-known actress who wrote a best seller about her amnesia of more than twenty years of an infantile trauma in which both her parents and siblings died in a fire at the family home.

References

Dupérey, A. (1992). *Le Voile noir*. Paris: Seuil.

Freud, S. (1900). *The Interpretation of Dreams*. S.E., 4–5. London: Hogarth.

Freud, S. (1915). The unconscious. S.E., 14. London: Hogarth, pp. 166–204.

Freud, S. (1924). The economic problem of masochism. S.E., 19. London: Hogarth, pp. 159–170.

Freud, S. (1950 [1895]). *A Project for a Scientific Psychology*. S.E., 1. London: Hogarth, pp. 295–397.

Grubrich-Simitis, I., et al. (2011). *Sei mein, wie ich mir's denke: Brautbriefe*. Frankfurt am Main: Fischer.

3　Tiredness

A masochism "in the feminine"

A conversation between women:

> "How are you?"
> "I'm exhausted, and you?"
> "I'm dead . . . What shall we do this evening?"
> "Let's go to the cinema. Before the film, we could pop over to
> Chantilly . . . There's a flea market . . .".

In Greek, instead of saying *morte*, we say πτῶμα (*ptoma*) . . . I am *corpse*. But the words are the same in English, *I am dead*, and in Spanish, *Muerta* . . .

At the level of the discourse, the women's tiredness is a mere observation: they refer to it as an old companion, but quickly pass on to something else . . . They live with their tiredness. Whether it is in life or in my daily practice, I have never heard a man speak in this way. If a man settles down on my couch and says, "I am dead", I am alarmed; if it is a woman, I wait to see what follows . . .

When I was younger and worked in centres catering for a population of ordinary people with "light" psychiatric troubles, I sometimes felt dizzy listening to the account of an ordinary day in the life of a simple, ordinary woman: waking up at six, getting three children of different ages dressed, including a baby; first to the nursery, then to school with the others, next the bus to the train or tube and work, a process that was later repeated in the reverse direction, followed by tea, and dinner . . . and finally some "quiet" ironing when everyone else had gone to bed.

"But you must be tired?" I would ask. "It's O.K." was a common answer; for these women did not come for a consultation because they were overworked; they came because of bereavements, phobias, anxieties, disappointments in love. Very early on, then, I developed the idea of feminine endurance.

Among the cohort of "depressions", tiredness was considered as an "abnormal" phenomenon and struggled against as an illness in itself; whereas, within the framework of the various psychopathological disorders, it was seen as belonging to a classical experience.

DOI: 10.4324/9781003197652-4

I wondered if this way of speaking about "their" tiredness and of living with it as a companion should be regarded as related to what is in the order of a "grievance", and consequently, of masochism.

It is difficult, I think, to tackle the question of "feminine tiredness" without referring to primary erotogenic masochism and its function as a "guardian of life", as Benno Rosenberg (2003) spoke of it. This quality of masochism is an existential dimension; it is what makes it possible to hold firm, to continue to invest interest in life, even when it is intolerable.

I am not going to impose on you a long detour in the meanders of "this accursed problem of masochism", the existence of which Ferenczi himself said raises a "vital question" for psychoanalytic theory.

For, while pleasure and suffering mingle and coincide, what becomes of the pleasure principle, which was hitherto regarded as the guardian of psychic life?

As he had been working on infantile psychosexuality ever since his *Three Essays on the Theory of Sexuality*, Freud (1905) was familiar with masochism as a clinical fact. He spoke about it but resisted recognising it as a primary phenomenon. He clearly did not want to make it a constituent of mental life.

It was not until twenty years later with "The economic problem of masochism" (Freud, 1924) that he was obliged to accept the idea of a primary masochism, leading him to undertake a radical re-examination of his theory, which had hitherto only been outlined. Indeed, up until 1920, Freud – who, moreover, followed Gustav Fechner – saw the pleasure principle as the foundation and regulating principle of mental functioning; that is to say, mental activity as a whole had the aim of avoiding unpleasure and procuring pleasure. But, for Freud, *unpleasure* was defined as tension caused by excitation, and *pleasure* as the reduction of this tension – a strictly economic definition that he was to call into question in 1920: "Pleasurable tensions exist" (exquisite pains).

This brings me back to the question of the feminine. Freud was not really concerned with this issue, and although he described a feminine masochism, it involved something else. But what I am proposing is the idea of a psychosexual difference, bearing in mind that anatomy, as well as the complex evolution of the feminine Oedipal configuration, favour the eroticisation in girls of the tension of excitation, whereas the path of discharge (namely the pleasure of reducing tensions) is more frequently used by men.

If the reader is ready to go along with my hypothesis, following the theory of Rosenberg, who regards primary masochism – binding destructivity – as the guardian of life, we can suppose that the cathexis of painful tension is "easier" or more "common" in women.

In this sense, it is permissible to think of tiredness as a painful tension; hence, the possibility of cathecting it without seeking immediately to evacuate it: "Be wise, O my tiredness, and keep me company".

I referred above to anatomy, but also the complex evolution of the feminine Oedipal configuration. Julia Kristeva (Kristeva & Clement, 2015) has spoken about this: the little girl turns away from her first love-object and chooses the father, whom she will have to renounce erotically in order to take possession of him through identification (Freud says this about boys); I believe this is a very important process in girls, because it is this identification that puts her on the side of action – of the symbolic, in Lacanian terms.

This is how, it seems to me, Julia Kristeva understands the two sides of the Oedipal configuration: it is increased psychic bisexuality in women, for whom the primary Oedipus is intensified by a secondary Oedipus.

Furthermore, the feminine superego is not easily constituted: it is the father as a seductive object, who is, at the same time, the bearer of the law. It is a more complex superego, which is dissolved in love. All these aspects also contribute to a more pronounced psychic bisexuality; paths of passage between one identificatory position and another are more frequent. The greater plasticity of the woman's body attests to this.

Women are psychic hermaphrodites: it is this flexibility that accounts for women's endurance. And yet, tired women exist . . . and pathologically tired women. The syndrome of chronic tiredness also affects women; as for fibromyalgia, it only affects women.

Fibromyalgia: a new illness consisting of painful tensions

Without tangible, organic causality, the symptoms of fibromyalgia remain mysterious and embarrassing for medical professionals. It raises nosographical controversies for many doctors. Some psychiatrists see hysterical manifestations in it. Pains and tiredness are compounded by other functional and vegetative symptoms, often accumulated, affecting all the systems. Finally, irritability, anxiety and diffuse anxieties, disorders of concentration and memory, not to mention insomnia, often lead to an inability to work or even to early retirement on health grounds. Drug-based therapeutics (tranquilizers and anti-depressants) do not provide improvement. Patients feel better when the pains diminish; on the other hand, tiredness persists and they then tend to complain even more about it.

Fibromyalgia is thus considered as a distinct entity resulting from a dysfunction of the systems that inhibit pain. Studies show that, in women with fibromyalgia, the threshold of pain is reduced. Peripheral sensitisation – which involves not only muscles but also tendons, ligaments and the skin – is amplified and generalised by central dysfunction. Some research studies have raised an epistemological difficulty; namely, the interweaving of pain and tiredness, where one can give rise to the other or result from it. The connection between the two is thought to be related to the sleep disorders highlighted in these patients.

Two particular characteristics emerge from consultations with patients suffering from fibromyalgia. The pains occur following a traumatic event that marks a change in the subject's life. Often, it is a bereavement, particularly concerning the loss of the mother, an emotional rupture or a failure in sentimental or professional life. The onset of crises occurs, in general, after the age of forty, which may indicate a focal point of libidinal and identificatory reorganisation, accentuated by obvious biological modifications in women. The second characteristic is based on the fact that the women concerned are always hyperactive, employing behavioural defences, and in particular, resorting to motor functioning. This hypertonicity is a feature of their professional life, which is demanding and requires a great deal of energy, bringing into play the requirements of a ferocious and unsatisfied ideal ego. Daily tasks, for example, are described as ordeals or competitions.

These women burn themselves up at work, as if they were responding to an internal injunction to always do more. They are in search of narcissistic validation and reassurance and feel that they are under a constant obligation to achieve results. This hypertonia finally exhausts the subject, who is caught in the trap of his or her own defence mechanisms, where the reduction of tensions is sought in action and the search for excitation, similar to the self-calming procedures described by psychosomatists (Michel Fain, Claude Smadja, Gérard Szwec).

Marina Papageorgiou (2003), a specialist for these patients, has described a particular configuration at the centre of the history of women suffering from fibromyalgia. During their childhood, they functioned as child therapists for their mother, and a particular distortion in the mother/daughter relationship can be observed. In one way or another, they were led to take care of a mother who was suffering mentally, but sometimes also physically, being either ill or disabled. The mother is in a state of physical dependence, but is described as courageous, rebellious and hyperactive both outside and inside the home – in spite of sometimes limited sensorimotor capacities – very demanding and a perfectionist. What dominates in the maternal figure is an excess of physical presence and a will to dominate.

In all cases, during their childhood, these women felt themselves to be morally and physically responsible for the mental and physical integrity of their mother.

An illness of rest due to the impossibility of relaxation

According to Pierre Marty (1980), object-relations are fixed early on by cathexes anchored in the sensorimotor sphere, depending on the responses of the mother and her capacity to ensure the somatopsychic instinctual integration of the child and to support the flow of stimuli in fantasy. Sometimes, the mother is unable to "let go" of the baby's body because she lacks a sufficient capacity for reverie, in such a way that her anxiety or her narcissism impede the infant's development; for example, in games and day-dreams. We can liken the non-reparative sleep and muscular hypervigilance of women with fibromyalgia to Michel Fain's theorisation on the need for a rhythm alternating between the cathexis and de-cathexis of the infant by the mother so that sleep, the guardian of the soma, can occur, with the corollary of dreaming as the guardian of sleep. This quality of the mother is linked to the "censorship of the woman-as-lover" (*censure de l'amante*) (Braunschweig & Fain, 1975), which brings into play the discontinuity between the mother's libido and the feminine libido of the mother-as-lover, who de-cathects her baby in order to rediscover erotic intimacy with her man. When things go well, the "censorship of the woman-as-lover" reinforces the narcissistic aims of the maternal function described by Marty.

In these patients, beyond non-reparative sleep, oneiric activity is reduced and dreams remain related to daytime activities. They do not provide any pleasure or satisfaction.

The story of Paulette

Paulette came to me at the age of fifty-eight. She was a tall and heavy Métis woman, though not obese or ungracious. She was sad and in despair, but her face sometimes lit up with a smile. She had been suffering from fibromyalgia for three years and was therefore on prolonged sick leave. Paulette had worked hard as a head nurse in a paediatrics department. Her illness appeared shortly after the retirement of a boss whom she had liked very much; she had been his "right hand" for thirty-five years. A few months earlier, she had also lost her brother, who had died in a car accident.

Her early childhood was marked by losses and upheavals. Born at the end of the war of an unknown father, she had been placed in a nursery – she did not know where. When she was five, her mother, who had since remarried, took her back again, and she lived for a few years with her family. She kept house and looked after her little brother, the son of her stepfather. Due to a move, she was once again placed in child care around the age of twelve. Her memories were vague, incomplete, full of gaps and uncertainties. Around the age of twenty, she met up again with her divorced mother in Paris. Paulette worked as a nursing auxiliary, did nursing studies and looked after her mother, whom she took care of mentally and materially.

When the patient decided to get married, her mother became depressed, fell ill and threatened to commit suicide. The young couple decided to live with her. They had no children – it was not a decision, but they took no medical steps in that direction. And then, as Paulette said to me, "It may be better like that . . . a three-room flat would've been small for four of us". In fact, the mother, who was depressive, bitter and ageing, assumed increasingly the place of a spoilt and capricious child. Neither Paulette nor her husband seemed to take umbrage. They complained about it when they found themselves alone together, but never called this cohabitation into question.

The sudden death of her brother upset this precarious equilibrium. This brother had stormy and difficult relations with his mother. He almost never saw her, called her a vampire, reproached Paulette for her weakness, but nonetheless remained the object of his mother's adoration. Paulette, who was very critical and jealous of this loved brother, told me that she had been saddened by his death, but "ravaged" by her mother's suffering in connection with it. For her mother, it was as if "a part of her body had been torn off". I took up this image, which I found intriguing, linking it up with the psychic separation from her boss, whose "right hand" she had been, and the painful burning sensations in her limbs due to her fibromyalgia. Shortly after, Paulette, who also found relief in painkillers, was to complain bitterly about how her pains had decreased; her extreme tiredness seemed to her to be even more overwhelming. I pointed out to her that, having lost her son, her mother had become even more of a weight for her to bear. This intervention inaugurated a period of anger, mixed with hateful reproaches directed towards her mother. Her mother's state deteriorated, moreover, and she demanded more and more attention and care. Paulette was extenuated. She did not sleep much and badly when she did; she used the vacuum cleaner on her knees, being too tired to stand on her legs.

Her head, which she said was empty at the beginning, was now too full. Everything was changing. Paulette tried to reconstitute her history; she imagined the father whom she knew nothing about, attributed her mother with a past as a prostitute, accused her of having prevented her from being a mother by putting herself in the place of a child. Paulette felt a bit better because she had finally succeeded in losing some weight.

Nevertheless, one day, she arrived carefully dressed and with light make-up.

"I wanted to be elegant for our last session", she told me. "I'm stopping because if I continue, I will end up putting my mother in a hospice, and I don't want to do that".

I was extremely moved and remained silent, thinking about the intense physical struggle that she had to continue to have with this burdensome mother, and with this father of whom she was beginning to dream without having been able to take possession of him through identification.

I wondered how she would cope with her mother's death. As if she had heard me, Paulette continued, "Perhaps I will come back one day . . . when . . .", and her sentence was left hanging.

By way of conclusion, I would like to put forward a hypothesis here whose value is essentially metaphorical. Let us take the mysterious nosographical entity of "fibromyalgia" as an illustration of one of the figures of feminine tiredness. The illness may be seen as the outcome of a misuse of bisexuality impeding the identificatory reversals that, in classical theory, make endurance possible in women.

Combined with this misuse are obviously the classical phenomena that provoke in both sexes the impossibility of resting: difficulties of regression and the extreme anti-cathexis of any kind of passivity . . .

These patients suffering from fibromyalgia strain and exhaust themselves in the unattainable quest of being both – and not successively – more efficient than the virile man whom they take as a model and, at the same time, the ideal daughter of a damaged mother, whom they carry and feel constantly obliged to repair.

References

Braunschweig, D., & Fain, M. (1975). *La Nuit, le jour. Essai psychanalytique sur le fonctionnement mental*. Paris: Presses Universitaires de France.

Freud, S. (1905). *Three Essays on the Theory of Sexuality. S.E.*, 7. London: Hogarth, pp. 123–243.

Freud, S. (1924). The economic problem of masochism. *S.E.*, 19. London: Hogarth, pp. 159–170.

Kristeva, J., & Clement, C. (2015). *Le Féminin et le Sacré*. Paris: Albin Michel.

Marty, P. (1980). *L'Ordre psychosomatique*. Paris: Payot.

Papageorgiou, M. (2003). L'insoutenable légèreté du corps de la mère. *Revue française de psychanalyse* 2(24): 127–144.

Rosenberg, B. (2003). Masochisme mortifère, masochisme gardien de vie. In: *Monograph of the Revue française de psychanalyse*. Paris: Presses Universitaires Françaises.

4   When masochism is lacking*

In the last chapter, I conjectured the existence of a "masochism in the femi-nine", distinct from the feminine masochism described by Freud. Depending on the psychosexual destiny of the little girl, this masochism in the feminine is constructed differently and permits greater tolerance to pain and to the frustrations of life in women. In theory, masochism and narcissism are to be conceptualised within a general conception of the drives.

Introduced in 1914, narcissism is part of instinctual drive life as devel-oped by Freud in the second and last theory of the drives, which opposes the life drives and the death drives, forces of binding/forces of unbinding. The primordial function of masochism is the fusion of the two antago-nistic drives. Primary narcissism and primary masochism coexist at the beginning of life and are indiscernible.

Benno Rosenberg (2003) elucidated this conjunction by suggesting that there is a libidinal part at the heart of this instinctual drive fusion that corre-sponds to primary narcissism. Thus, any decrease in narcissistic capital would immediately have an influence on the constitution of masochism; that is, on the fusion between the life drive and the drive of unbinding/destruction.

What Rosenberg calls the "primary erotogenic masochistic nucleus of the ego" is the primary fusion of the libido with the death drive within the ego in its very constitution. This work of fusion forms the ego of the child. This theoretical notion is very pertinent and makes it possible to describe the economic movements between the narcissistic cathexes and the strength or weakness of primary erotogenic masochism.

The primary erotogenic masochistic nucleus, described by Rosenberg, is a fundamental conception for psychoanalysis and particularly crucial in psychosomatic clinical practice, where the masochistic cathexis of illness can either be seriously absent or become one of the factors of recovery.

In run of the mill clinical work, many patients presenting narcissistic deficiencies are eaten away by "negative" narcissism, so well-defined by

* This chapter was first published in 2010 under the title "Petites marques du corps" in the *Revue française de psychosomatique* ("Corps Marqués"), 38: 7–15.

DOI: 10.4324/9781003197652-5

André Green (2001), which is present in place of a positive narcissism – the "cement of the ego".

In the 1960s, Herbert Rosenfeld (1971) began to describe a destructive form of narcissism, for which he established a classification: "narcissistic patients with protective shells", "thin skinned" narcissistic patients, the syndrome of arrogance, and finally, narcissistic patients who mutilate themselves, presenting an extreme danger. Although they are primarily descriptive, Rosenfeld's descriptions still seem to me to be pertinent.

In André Green's work (1999, 2001), on the other hand, the conception of "negative narcissism" is the cornerstone of a complex and original theoretical edifice.

My concern here is above all to argue that the failures of narcissism are always linked to the failure of the work of the fusion of the drives by primary erotogenic masochism. We can therefore speak of a gradient, N/M.

The narcissism of small differences

Thinking about the marked body leads us inevitably to reflect on tattooing, piercing and other more or less extreme practices. Among the voluntary markings that the subject inflicts on himself, I would also include certain much more trivial particularities such as a moustache, a kiss curl, a hairstyle – a characteristic that is cathected as a "label" – "a distinctive mark" – condensing the whole personality, the quintessence of that particular individual's being in the world.

There are women who cannot resolve themselves to cut their hair. How many times have I heard: "My hair on my back, or my pony tail, that's me". The same is true for small, tiny physical defects: a bump on the nose, a slight squint, a beauty spot, a blemish. This had not escaped Freud's notice, who spoke of a "narcissism of minor differences". Curiously, this expression appeared in his article "The taboo of virginity" (Freud, 1918) following reflections on the differences between the sexes. In it, Freud cites Ernest Crawley, an English anthropologist who had written *The Mystic Rose: a Study of Primitive Marriage* (Crawley, 1902).

In a language that differs somewhat from that of psychoanalysts, Crawley had identified a notion that he called a "taboo of personal isolation". Minor differences between people who are otherwise fairly similar are held to be the source of feelings of strangeness and hostility that are so common in human beings. Freud subsequently refers to the narcissistic rejection of femininity by men and the taboo of virginity that confronts them, among other things with the horror of blood, while a woman is subject to defloration, which is a narcissistic injury for her integrity.

Freud returned to the narcissism of minor differences in 1921 in Chapter Six of *Group Psychology and the Analysis of the Ego* (Freud, 1921), then in 1930 in Chapter Five of *Civilization and its Discontents* (Freud, 1930), and finally in 1939 in *Moses and Monotheism* (Freud, 1939). The reflections he derived from this study are fascinating, while their sociological, anthropological and philosophical interest goes well beyond strictly psychoanalytic considerations.

I propose to examine here this singular narcissism by the "small end of the telescope". A trait, a detail, a particularity marked on the subject's own body sometimes seems to concentrate for this subject his specificity – his humanity – and to distinguish him from others. What, for example, can a moustache – his moustache – represent for an individual X or Y?

Many years ago, I was very intrigued by reading the novel by Emmanuel Carrère (1988) titled *The Moustache*.

A man in his early forties, who was accomplished and quite happy, without children, but clearly very much in love with his wife, had worn a moustache for such a long time that he could no longer recall what his face looked like when it was clean-shaven. He invested a very particular interest in his moustache and had developed real shaving rites. It was in the evening, in his bath, with a whisky placed on the edge of the bathtub, where there were also well-lit mirrors, that he devoted almost sacred attention to his moustache.

This moment of intimacy with himself is described by the writer as "a moment of relaxation organized with care". A psychoanalyst would speak of a turning round of narcissism onto his own person.

One evening, when the couple was due to have dinner with friends, he asked his wife, "What would you say if I shaved off my moustache?" Probably distracted, instead of saying as usual, "I like you with it", she replied: "That might be a good idea", then went out to buy something while reminding him of the time at which they had to leave. From this moment on, the reader senses that something inevitable is going to happen. "He" – he is never referred to in any other way – shuts himself in the bathroom, shaves a first time at length and carefully. He plays with the idea of shaving off his moustache to surprise his wife. Besides, she was always changing her hairstyle without asking him. We can sense that he is caught in a conflict of a narcissistic order. Should he take her at her word and be strong? But, at what price, he had no idea as yet. Or did his provocations risk being tinged with the colour of adolescent revolt? In any case, he would be castrated, but preferred to ignore it. There was a lot at stake, but "he" was not yet conscious of it. He treated it all as a joke.

When he had finished the usual shaving ritual, during which he would care lovingly for his moustache, he impulsively took the fatal decision to eradicate it, to sacrifice it. He began trimming it:

> It immediately occurred to him that this clump of hair might clog the bathtub drain . . . He took the toothbrush glass which he placed on the bathtub rim; then precariously poised, he leaned toward the mirror and went about trimming off the bulk of his moustache. The hair fell to the bottom of the glass in compact little tufts, which were very black against the whitish tartar deposit.
>
> (Carrère, 1988, p. 4)

Looking in the mirror, he thought, somewhat surprised: "Not great", identifying himself with the way his wife would be seeing him. He was impatient to have her reaction.

Up to this point, whether he is a psychoanalyst or not, the reader can follow the situation easily. After, the narrative becomes infinitely more enigmatic.

Agnes, his wife, did not notice anything. At first, he thought that she was just paying him back and pretending artfully not to notice anything. "Two can play at that game", he thought; he admired his wife, she was such a good actress. He stood firm too, but when the couple of friends they visited in the evening also seemed not to notice anything, his anxiety increased. He dealt with it by imagining a conspiracy of silence: perhaps Agnes had warned them by telephone; the word had got round. It was a joke that was going a bit too far for his liking.

When they were going home in the car, he implored Agnes, "Please stop. I'm asking you to stop it". She didn't understand or pretended not to understand.

The reader is now also disturbed and anxious. Who is mad? Is he a delusional mythomaniac? Is she suffering from a negative hallucination concerning the past?

> "What's this story about a moustache?"
> "Agnès, I shaved it off. It's not important, it'll grow back. Look at me, Agnes" . . .
> "You know very well that you never had a moustache. Stop it, please . . . Please, you're scaring me, stop it".
>
> (ibid., p. 24)

The next day, in the middle of the night, he could not sleep and was thinking about the dustbin, about the little plastic bag which must still have the remains of his moustache in it. He hoped that Agnes had not had time to *get rid of the evidence*. He continued to think it was a collective prank, whose sadistic dimension amazed him. We went down to where the trash cans were and started to rummage through them frantically. He found all sorts of things and also some hair scattered all over the place, some of which he collected in the palm of his hand. He woke Agnes up and showed it to her. She told him he was crazy.

"And this?" he said, opening the palm of his hand, as if to convince himself, "What do you call this?" (p. 49).

This was the beginning of a descent into the hell of madness. Armed with his identity card, on which he visibly had a moustache, he wandered in the streets of Paris asking strangers if they recognised him on the photo. He feigned being blind and stopped a young woman, holding out his papers to her; she confirmed that it was indeed him. He insisted on asking her to tell him if he is wearing a moustache, like in the picture. She started to feel afraid.

The following day, he had dinner at a restaurant with Agnes; he was very concerned about his wife's mental health and so tried to give the impression of being light and detached. He paid by check and had to show his identity card. She took hold of it and, to prove to him that the moustache in the photo had recently been added with a magic marker, she scraped the document with her nails and then with a little razor. "Paralyzed, he watched her do it, removing from his upside-down face fine black particles scraping until the space between his nose and his mouth had become, not grey, like the rest of the photo, but a grainy slashed-up white" (p. 77).

"He" felt more and more shocked: in the strict sense of the term, he was in a traumatic state. After some increasingly crazy peregrinations, it occurred to him that he had to leave. He had to get away from his crazy wife who was, in addition, probably dangerous. On a sudden impulse, he had himself driven to Roissy airport and bought a ticket for Hong Kong that did not require a visa.

In Hong Kong the pathological wandering that is well known to psychiatrists began. Days passed, during which he went through a succession of mental states ranging from persecution to depression to cosmic delusion. Yet he knew that he was of sound mind:

> He wasn't crazy. Neither were Agnes, Jerome or the others. It was just that the order of the world had been thrown out of whack, it was both abominable and discreet, it had passed unnoticed by everyone but him, which put him in the position of being the only witness to the crime, which consequently had to be fought. . . . He should make Agnes understand this necessity . . . his disappearance was a vital obligation.
>
> (pp. 146–147)

He wandered aimlessly, rode the ferries and gradually became a tramp, but continued to shave twice a day, while allowing his moustache to grow again. One day, he returned to the hotel and learnt that Agnes was in his room. She talked to him as if nothing had happened, as if they were travelling together or on holiday. The reader once again asks himself: Which of them is mad? Or is she trying to drug him in order to repatriate him and get treatment for him?

In any case, he replied in the same tone and simply asked if he could use the bathroom. He locked the door, and standing in front of the mirror, "started in on the moustache": he cut out the triangle of flesh where, according to him, there was once a moustache. He mutilated himself where the moustache had been, indicated by a hole in his flesh; he marked himself permanently and looked at himself. Then, when the pain became intolerable, he continued and cut his throat.

I am familiar with the recourse to literature treated as a clinical document, and it has often seemed to me to be very enriching. Here, the example is both tragic and extreme. It came to my mind associatively. I had in mind the theme of Volume 15 of the *Revue française de psychanalyse* in Autumn 1999, devoted to pain, and was thinking of writing about tattooing when I saw a young woman for a consultation who presented serious states of depersonalisation. She then ran away, or rather disappeared for forty-eight hours, following a minor aesthetic operation.

A beauty spot

O was an American student in Paris for one year. Having done art studies in a university of North Carolina, she was now preparing a Ph.D., which required her to do some research in Parisian galleries, and she was taking advantage of her stay to learn French. She shared the rent of an apartment with another American student.

O described herself as happy and without difficulties, saying that she came from a well-off family in an aristocratic milieu of the South that had always loved and protected her. She had two brothers in the United States whom she loved, who were brilliant students and finishing their university studies. She explained to me that she had always been considered as the "little princess", who was more than pretty, quite a good student, lively and playful, not at all "the kind to be anxious or depressed".

As I was listening to her, I had some difficulty in matching the picture she described of herself with the defeated and terrorised young woman who was sitting in front of me. She had been referred to me by a psychiatrist who had seen her and put her on drugs. He had wondered about hospitalising her in a clinic and wanted to have my opinion. The alternative was for me to see her three or four times while waiting for her parents to come and collect her and take her back to the States. Their trip was planned and Dr N. was in contact with them.

O had a beauty spot that was bigger than a fly, approximately half a centimeter in diameter, on her right cheek, near the nostril. She had always had it, she said tearfully, "ever since her birth". She had Venetian blond hair and a lot of freckles and saw her American dermatologist every year for a routine check-up. In Paris, friends of her parents recommended a dermatologist to her, whom she went to see for no other reason than to "check her beauty spots".

Far from reassuring her as his American counterpart had done, the French doctor called into question the benign nature of the beauty spot, talked about the risk of a melanoma, and said she had no time to lose. In short, he scared her and persuaded her to let him operate on it himself, especially as he was also a plastic surgeon. Two days later, she was admitted to a private clinic, where she underwent a relatively important operation, under a general anaesthetic, since it involved eradicating the "beauty spot" without leaving *a hole in her cheek*.

O said nothing about this to either her family or friends, because she wanted to be courageous and worthy. She told her flat mate that she had to undergo a "minor dental procedure". She only told them later about the danger of cancer and the swift decision she had taken. She was delighted to have remained so calm and admired her own maturity. She thought that her parents would be proud of her. She could already see herself telling the story in a serious but light tone that she had always admired in the women on her mother's side, who were capable of remaining ladylike in the worst moments.

In this connection, she mentioned her grandmother, a widow and very beautiful woman who was eighty, continued to travel alone, and knew India like the back of her hand. This grandmother was from a big, Southern family and had campaigned for the election of Barack Obama. O mentioned in passing that she also had a beauty spot on the right cheek, but higher up and near the cheekbone.

This account was interspersed with tears, uncontrolled sobbing and short silences, during which she wrung her hands and writhed as if she could not find any position that was comfortable for her. I thought she looked pale; and she had big bags under her eyes. She had also lost weight, she told me; she had difficulty sleeping and eating, in spite of the drugs. She made me think of a child lost in a crowd, a child who was afraid of not finding her family again.

I only met O three times. It was not a matter of giving her interpretations. I had two aims: to hear her anxiety while trying, with her, to link it up with representations and to make her see the interest of doing a long-term analysis on her return to the United States. My fear was that the episode would be quickly "closed" and suppressed. During our second meeting three days later, O gave me more precise details about her meeting with the surgeon/dermatologist. She felt terrible for having trusted him immediately. He spoke English without an accent and had been attentive and paternal. In other words, without putting it like this, she said she had been seduced by an Oedipal substitute. He had told her that she was in danger, that she could trust him, but also that she would be "even more beautiful without this spot on her cheek". But this physical particularity was a kind of bond with her idealised maternal grandmother who had "almost the same" thing. So, he cut the maternal line for her in her fantasies, which was considered dangerous due to the verdict of malignity.

In addition, he had mentioned a "hole in the cheek" which he would fill. Now, although she had not taken notice of this formulation during the medical interview, it was precisely this hole that she thought she could see under the bandages the day after the operation. She had had a full-blown panic attack and had been put on a drip, which sent her to sleep for forty-eight hours. On waking up, she was in a state of depersonalisation, obsessed by the *idea of a hole under her bandages*.

She clearly seemed to have fantasies of being raped but the surgeon and nurses, who were probably very alarmed, suggested transferring her to a psychiatric clinic and then called a psychiatrist to her bedside. He understood that she was suffering from acute hysterical symptoms rather than psychosis. He visited her daily until she could leave the clinic and then referred her to me. This remarkable psychiatrist had been very worried, after she had left the clinic, by the fact that her flat mate R. had told him that O had disappeared for nearly eighteen hours.

O could not recall what she had done. She knew that she had returned in the early morning, by which time R. had already called the doctor and was about to go to the police. She had probably wandered through Paris in a "hysterical twilight state", as psychiatrists once used to say. I said to her:

"Perhaps you were searching for your grandmother, who had the same beauty spot. It is as if you had lost your ties with her since this man took out this mark".

O seemed taken aback, looked at me for a while and the smiled. When she was little, she had always wanted this particular grandma; it's true, she had looked for her. Everywhere.

When we met for the last time, O seemed replenished; she had just seen Dr N.: "He was brilliant!" I nodded.

She told me that she had had the idea that one day she might get a "tattoo of her beauty spot", once her cheek had fully healed. Without saying anything, I thought: *to erase all the traces of the crime*. And this was when I thought of the novel. She noticed my puzzlement.

"Do you think I should do an analysis first?", she asked. I answered very simply that, in general, I thought it was better first to try and understand and then to act as a second step. O remained silent for a long time and then explained to me that my suggestion was not in line with the family model, but mainly paternal, according to which you must act or else you are a loser.

Nevertheless, her grandmother and even her mother were a bit different – "more European". Moreover, O had already told me about her grandmother's long trips abroad and to India.

I cannot stop myself from saying that *I would like O to do a good analysis*, because she has the psychic means to do so.

My resolute optimism for this very young woman, whom I found beautiful and likeable, was tempered by the reminiscence of the novel by Emmanuel Carrère, which I had recently re-read. How can a moustache or a beauty spot take on such importance to the point of representing a danger of a narcissistic cataclysm for the subject?

The Oedipal organisation and its outcome play a decisive role. We know nothing about the past of "he" in the novel. But O revealed very quickly that she had a history going back over three generations. It can easily be surmised that we are dealing here with present states of mind, on which we know nothing as yet about the impact of past events. But it is not of the two stages of castration or trauma that I want to speak about here, but of a phenomenon in the order of *a "stasis" of the narcissistic libido, in which the small marks on the subject's body can be concentrated.*

Narcissism of minor differences? I am aware that I am giving an extension to the Freudian notion; nonetheless, it is a similar phenomenon, where a mark on the body becomes a "taboo" owing to the narcissistic cathexis of it – a cathexis that transforms this mark into the guarantor of the individual's narcissistic integrity.

Do we not speak of "birth marks" or "trademarks" which cannot be touched? A taboo is a taboo, and its transgression can lead to the disorganisation of identity and death.

Freud saw libidinal stasis as an economic process that could be at the origin of the onset of neurosis or psychosis, but classically it is an accumulation of libido in intrapsychic formations. Is it not possible to imagine the same process, the same "stasis" accumulating in places on the subject's own body that are highly cathected?

Freud (1915) examines the withdrawals of libido into the body in illness and hypochondria. He compares them and puts forward the hypothesis that hypochondria is the third actual neurosis. I wonder if *these small marks* I am talking about were not initially the object of a hypochondriacal cathexis. This would also confer on them a status similar to that of the erotogenic zones and they would then be the vehicle of a life narcissism, but also a death narcissism.

References

Carrère, E. (1988/1986). *The Moustache,* trans. Lanie Goodman. London: Penguin, Random House.

Crawley, E. (1902). *The Mystic Rose: A Study of Primitive Marriage.* London: Macmillan.

Freud, S. (1915). *Instincts and their Vicissitudes. S.E.,* 14. London: Hogarth, pp. 111–140.

Freud, S. (1918). *The Taboo on Virginity. S.E.,* 11. London: Hogarth, pp. 193–208.

Freud, S. (1921). *Group Psychology and the Analysis of the Ego. S.E.,* 18. London: Hogarth, pp. 65–144.

Freud, S. (1930). *Civilization and Its Discontents. S.E.,* 21. London: Hogarth, pp. 59–145.

Freud, S. (1939). *Moses and Monotheism. S.E.,* 23. London: Hogarth, pp. 3–137.

Green, A. (1999/1993). *The Work of the Negative,* trans. Andrew Weller. London: Free Association Books.

Green, A. (2001/1991). *Life Narcissism, Death Narcissism.* London: Free Association Books.

Rosenberg, B. (2003). Masochisme mortifère, masochisme gardien de vie. In: *Monograph of the Revue française de psychanalyse.* Paris: Presses Universitaires Françaises.

Rosenfeld, H. (1971). A clinical approach to the psychoanalytic theory of the life and death instincts: An investigation into the aggressive aspects of narcissism. *International Journal of Psychoanalysis* 52(2): 169–178. Available on https:// pubmed.ncbi.nlm.nih.gov/?term=%22Int+J+Psychoanal%22%5Bjour%5D

5   Thinking: an act of the flesh*

Chapter XLVIII of Tertullian's *Apologeticum*[1] is titled "De Carnis Ressurectio". It contains this striking statement: "Thinking is an act of the flesh". Tertullian was a Carthaginian whose date of birth is uncertain, though situated around 160 A.D., and the peak of his writing activity unfolded between 193 and 217 A.D. He is described as having an ardent and passionate nature. He had studied law, medicine and philosophy, and was immensely erudite. He had had a pagan background, enjoyed circus games, practised wrestling and enjoyed the pleasures of the flesh. He entered into his pleasures and his studies with passion, and no doubt sensuality, too, qualities which, after his conversion around the age of thirty, he put to the service of defending the Christian faith.

"De Carnis Ressurectio" is very interesting and unusual because, in my view, it is in keeping with a philosophical monism that was both extremely rare at that time and very different from the usual dualism of Christianity. Tertullian's argument is built on refuting the idea that the body is the sole perishable envelope of the soul. He defends the idea of a whole.

Speaking of the resurrection, he writes:

> The soul alone cannot suffer at all without a material substance, that is, the flesh; and because souls have incurred whatever generally it is their due to suffer from God's judgement, not without the flesh within which all their actions were performed" (*"non sine carne meruerunt, intra quam omnia egerunt"*.
>
> (Tertullian, XLVIII, 121)

This view of a psyche moved and transformed by its body was visionary in the second century A.D. and very similar to Freud's (1900) affirmation: "Thought is after all nothing but a substitute for a hallucinatory wish . . . nothing but a wish can set our mental apparatus at work" (p. 567).

---

* This chapter was first published in 2015 under the title "Psychisation du corps, incarnation de la pensée" in *Monographies et débats de psychanalyse* (La pensée: Approche psychanalytique), pp. 31–46.

DOI: 10.4324/9781003197652-6

In one of my earlier articles (Aisenstein & Dreyfus, 1995), I argued, with my co-author, that Freud and the discovery of psychoanalysis could not have happened if Spinoza had not posited the unity of substance and defended the notion of "materialist monism", thereby opposing the body/mind dualism that had dominated Western philosophy. Psychoanalysis, in fact, could only find its place within a monistic current, which is illustrated by the description of hysterical conversion (I nonetheless continue to be amazed by this oneness anticipated fifteen centuries earlier by a Christian preacher).

In Freud's work, the body is present from the outset through sexuality, and the concepts of desire and drive are essential for tackling the central points; namely, the question of the somatic origins of thought, the transition from the sensory dimension to affect, and then to desexualised thought.

As psychosomaticians, we work with patients whose discourse is not – or is no longer – *alive*; it is cut off from its instinctual drive roots. These are often patients who build their lives against desire. I will begin, therefore, by reflecting on the notion of desire in Freud's work, in the light of the concept of primary erotogenic masochism.

Desire, waiting, thought

As I described in Chapter 2, "The birth of desire", Freud outlined his theory of desire on the basis of observations of the new-born child, who creates *memory images* associating experiences of satisfaction with the desired object. These experiences leave traces in the form of *unpleasurable affects* and states of wishing (*états de désir*), characterised by internal tension followed by release. The baby passes from the vital need for milk to the mother, who gives her breast to him.

Only psychic work permits the transition from need to desire. This transition implies that the distressing excitation is alleviated by an experience of satisfaction that is memorised and creates an attraction to the object. This movement towards the object is called "desire". Desire arises from need; the recognition of desire becomes the basis of recognition of the object and thereby of the subject who, henceforth, is necessarily a "desiring subject". Let me cite again Freud's *The Interpretation of Dreams*:

> All this activity of thought is merely constitutes a roundabout path to wish-fulfilment, which has been made necessary by experience. Thought is after all nothing but a substitute for a hallucinatory wish; and it is self-evident that dreams must be wish-fulfilments, since nothing but a wish can set our mental apparatus at work.
>
> (Freud, 1900, p. 567)

Desire is therefore at the basis of psychic work and thought.

At the risk of repeating myself, I remain convinced that the transition from the vital need to desire – which implies waiting, psychic work and thought – remains incomprehensible without the conception of primary erotogenic masochism, which binds the contradictory drive impulses in the child's ego.

Due to the binding of the libido and the death drive, a movement that unbinds and immobilises, primary masochism makes possible the integration of the capacity for waiting.

Here, the mother's psychic work is fundamental. She must know how to help the infant to accept waiting. Benno Rosenberg had invented the term "fusing/entangling mother" (*mère intricante*). I would prefer to say: a "mother who creates a work of fusion/entanglement".

The concept of primary masochism is indispensable here because, if waiting is to be tolerable, it must be "masochistically cathected". Rosenberg (2003) showed this brilliantly in his *Masochisme mortifère, Masochisme gardien de vie*, a monograph published in that year by the *Revue française de psychanalyse*. The infant must gradually be led to understand that there is also pleasure to be had in waiting, even if it is painful. This cathexis of delay is at the basis of desire: *I think and I imagine the pleasure to come.*

The structure of desire is masochistic in essence; for desire is inconceivable without giving up immediate satisfaction and without cathecting waiting. I could give many examples of how this cathexis of waiting occurs: *The Princess of Clèves, Anna Karenin, In Search of Lost Time, The Odyssey*, and so on.

In this context, it is to the young Freud that I would like to return, and more precisely, to the exchange of letters referred to earlier in Chapter 2. As we can read in this epistolary volume, there is desire in love, and there is dreaming, thinking and even pleasure in these anticipatory thoughts. Theories of hallucination, of desire and representation (of words and things) are already present in embryo in the exchanges between Freud and Martha.

In Freud, there is no explicit theory of thought, or of unconscious perception, moreover, which nonetheless contributes to the dream-thoughts. Yet he wrote in 1890:

> The affects in the narrower sense are, it is true, characterized by a quite special connection with somatic processes; but, strictly speaking, all mental states, including those that we usually regard as "processes of thought" are to some degree "affective", and not one of them is without its physical manifestations or is incapable of modifying somatic processes. Even when a person is quietly engaged in thinking in a string of "ideas", there are a constant series of excitations corresponding to the contents of these ideas, which are discharged into the smooth or striated muscles.
>
> Freud (1905a [1890], p. 288)

I have always found this early article deeply moving. For me, it is a visionary text because it contains in germ not only the entire theory of the drive – a boundary concept between the body and the mind – but also the theory of the Paris school of psychosomaticians.

On this same page, a few lines further, Freud explains how the perception by a sensitive subject of the somatic manifestations of another person and even "certain striking, and ostensibly 'supernatural' phenomena can be explained by this means. Thus, what is known as 'thought-reading' may be explained by small, involuntary muscular movements carried out by the 'medium'" (ibid.).

In this last sentence, I can also see the bases for a reflection on a theme that is dear to me – that of unconscious perception in the dream-thoughts – and moreover, on the question of the countertransference.

Unconscious perception

Freud never developed a theory of unconscious perception.[2] It nevertheless exists implicitly in his work and underpins the theory of dreams. Without this theory, the whole of Chapter VII in *The Interpretation of Dreams* (Freud, 1900) would be strictly incomprehensible, and in particular, the sentences written above. Latent thoughts consist of perceptions that remain unconscious in the waking state.

A diagnostic dream

> A woman patient had to make a long car journey. The night before she was due to leave, she had a nightmare that woke her up: in the rear mirror she saw that the back of her car was on fire. She told me that she made the journey the following day without thinking any further about it. When she was about 240 miles from Paris, she saw in the mirror that black smoke was rising up, most probably from the exhaust pipe. Alerted, she called for help. The garage mechanic who examined her vehicle said it could have caught fire if she had not stopped immediately and asked her if she had not heard in recent days "a little noise coming from the rear end". Having no interest in mechanics, she had not heard anything. Yet her dream was clearly a "diagnostic dream" containing the "hypochondriacal magnification" of dreams described by Freud.
>
> Freud (1917, p. 223)

In clinical work, part of the analyst's unconscious and preconscious countertransference is made up of counter-perceptions of that part of the patient's transference that is least known to him. Equally, some patients react violently to the slightest signs of their analyst's moods. Here, I fully agree with Lacan when he says that the countertransference is the other side of the transference.

The transference therefore includes the subject and the psychoanalyst in a continuous unconscious flow.

Countertransference

A patient arrived for his 3 o'clock session and I had just got back feeling exhausted after a long morning in the Centre. He began telling me in great detail about the delightful meal he had had in a top restaurant. I was tired and noticed that I felt slightly nauseous. At first, I attributed it to the fact that I had not eaten anything since the evening before and to a stormy session with a young schizophrenic patient whom I had had to hospitalise once again. This young woman moved me deeply and I was very concerned about her. The patient stopped talking and then said suddenly: "It's strange, but I'm feeling sick".

The unconscious perception by my patient of my envy, probably out of hate, of his enjoyable and luxurious lunch, helped me to understand the meaning of this nausea.

These typical phenomena of unconscious perception are at the heart of the transference and exist in every analysis. They are discreet in classical analyses where the putting into language and play of ideas are facilitated by associations, but take on importance in the technique of "more difficult" treatments.

The question of thought in the Freudian corpus

From 1890 to 1918

As André Green pointed out on many occasions, there is no theory of thought in Freud's work. Thought and thinking are not meta-psychological categories. It could be argued, however, that thought was his major preoccupation. Symptoms, neurotic (obsessions, phobias, etc.) and psychotic (delusions) appear to the phenomenologist to be disturbances or alterations of thought, which comprises judgment. Freud assumes that desire is the motor of psychic work which involves thought.

Freud substitutes Descartes' *Cogito ergo sum* with "I desire, therefore I am", just as he replaces Cartesian dualism by drive dualism within a monistic body/mind conception.

In fact, it is thought processes, their origin and their vicissitudes, that concern Freud more than thought itself. In 1893, he wrote the preliminary communication of the "Project for a scientific psychology" (Freud, 1950 [1895]), in which he links thought processes to memory and external reality, but above all to perception. The *Studies on Hysteria* (Freud, 1895) and then "The aetiology of hysteria" (Freud, 1896) demonstrate the specifically sexual origin of hysterical and neurotic symptoms in general.

At the same time, we can follow the path that leads in small steps to qualifying excitation – it becomes "sexual" and no longer somatic and diffuse – then to giving it a vectorisation, and finally, to a model of mental work.

In the *Three Essays on Sexuality*, Freud (1905b) began to conceive infantile sexuality, and thus the drive, as a dynamic mental process anchored in the body and desperately in search of an object. The concept of the drive became a meta-psychological category. The child's sexual curiosity is seen from the angle of an urge for investigation, forming the foundations of epistemophilia.

It is particularly interesting to observe how Freud always keeps hold of the guiding thread of the psychosexual. In "Leonardo da Vinci and a memory of his childhood" (Freud, 1910) offers us a reading of artistic sublimation in connection with sexuality. One year later, "Formulations on the two principles of mental functioning" (Freud, 1911) is the first – and only – text in which Freud gives a definition of thought in the waking state in relation to the pleasure principle and the reality principle:

> Thinking was endowed with characteristics that made it possible for the mental apparatus to tolerate an increased tension of stimulus while the process of discharge was postponed. *It is essentially an experimental kind of acting, accompanied by displacement of relatively small quantities of cathexis together with less expenditure (discharge) of them. For this purpose the conversion of freely displaceable cathexes into 'bound' cathexes was necessary, and this was brought about by means of raising the level of the whole cathectic process.*
>
> (Freud, 1911, p. 221, my emphasis)

It is probable that thought was unconscious in origin insofar as it "went beyond mere ideational presentations and was directed to the relations between impressions of objects, and that it did not acquire further qualities, perceptible to consciousness, until it became connected with verbal residues" (ibid.). Although it is rooted in the sexual under the aegis of pleasure, thought evolves under the principle of the reality-principle.

In the years that followed, Freud sought to clarify and explore more deeply the theoretical hypotheses on which his psychoanalytic system might be founded. In 1915, he wrote the five articles that make up the *Papers on Metapsychology*. In order to stick closely to the question of the body and thought, I am going to focus on "Instincts and their vicissitudes" (Freud, 1915).

The concept of the drive is fundamental, and Freud seeks to give it a content by approaching it from different angles, the first of which is physiology. "Let us imagine ourselves", he writes,

> in the situation of an almost entirely helpless living organism, as yet unoriented in the world, which is receiving stimuli in its nervous substance. This organism will very soon be in a position to make a first distinction. . . . On the one hand, it will be aware of stimuli which can be avoided by muscular action (flight); these it ascribes to an external world. On the other hand, it will also be aware of stimuli against which such action is of no avail and whose character of constant pressure persists in spite of it. These stimuli are the signs of an internal world, the evidence of instinctual needs.
>
> (Freud, 1915, p. 119)

The drives force the nervous system of the human being to give up its ideal intention of keeping stimuli at bay: *"We may therefore well conclude that* instincts . . . *are the true motive forces behind the advances that have led the nervous system, with its unlimited capacities to its present high level of development"* (p. 120, my emphasis). It is with this statement that Freud introduces the assumption of the "demand for representation" that I have already defended elsewhere (Aisenstein, 2010). Furthermore, he foresees here the whole problem of sublimation.

A little further on, we find his famous definition:

> If now we apply ourselves to considering mental life from a *biological* point of view, an "instinct" appears to us as a concept on the frontier between the mental and the somatic, as the psychical representative of the stimuli originating from within the organism and reaching the mind, as a measure of the demand made upon the mind for work in consequence of its connection with the body.
>
> (Freud, 1915, pp. 121–122)

Although psychoanalysis existed before the concept of the drive, I think that here, there is a before and an after in Freud's thought – a radical caesura. Freud was a neurologist by training and not a psychiatrist: building the concept of the drive was the only way for him to take account simultaneously of biology and neurophysiology, on the one hand, and of subjective experience, which includes affects and thought processes, on the other.

It is clear that the *demand comes from the body* which imposes on the mind a *measurable amount of work*, which I would say is indispensable for its protection and thus for its survival. Green (1999) has proposed a fine formulation:

> The psyche is, so to speak, worked by the body, worked in the body. . . . The body demands work from the mind (elaboration comes from labour). But this demand for work cannot be accepted in its raw state. It must be decoded if the mind is to respond to the demand of the body which, in the absence of any response, will increase its demands in force and in number.
>
> (p. 170)

Without an adequate response from the mind that is unable to provide representations, the drive is degraded and returns to the state of diffuse somatic excitation.

From 1915 to 1938

Announced subtly in "Leonardo da Vinci and a memory of his childhood" (Freud, 1910), the text "On narcissism: An introduction" was published in

1914 (Freud, 1914). I have always been intrigued by the prior appearance of the concept of narcissism, since, in 1915, Freud wrote the five principal articles that make up the *Papers in Metapsychology*. I have imagined that, seeing the significance of this article, Freud had, as it were, kept it in abeyance in order to reconsider its impact on his existing theoretical considerations. This text is fundamental for several reasons that concern the question of thought. It announces ineluctably the second drive theory, and consequently, the change of topography in 1923. Moreover, it seems unquestionable that narcissism plays a role in the cathexis of thought which has its roots in the sexual and remains unthinkable without a referring to narcissism.

In the introduction to *Life Narcissism, Death Narcissism*, Green (2000a) speaks of a "parenthesis in Freud" concerning narcissism. For my part, I would say a "period of abeyance" while waiting for the turning-point of 1920, as if Freud had not yet evaluated all the clinical and theoretical implications of the introduction of narcissism into the theory of the drives.

Freud does not seem to have envisaged the relations between narcissism and thought; for him, narcissism was a "state" and not a "structure", as it was for Green. Green's work elucidated and gave more depth to the metapsychology, and he showed how much the organisation of primary narcissism is at work in the construction of subjectivity.

In Freud's work, it is essentially the second drive theory that places emphasis on thought processes. Indeed, by substituting the first drive opposition between sexuality and self-preservation with the opposition between the libido and the death drive, Freud overcame a sterile debate (sexuality can be self-preservative and deadly) and he posited the existence of two drives – binding and unbinding – which define thought processes.

In the *Organon*,[3] Aristotle (385–322 B.C.) laid down the foundations of modern logic by dealing with a variety of questions. The writings that received the general title "Organon" (meaning "instrument, tool, organ") are an initiation to his scientific and philosophical texts. It is a collection of his six works, *Categories, On Interpretation* (analysis of statements), *Prior Analytics, Posterior Analytics* (the theory of syllogism and demonstration which depend on logic in the strict sense), *Topics* (the theory of argumentation) and *On Sophisticated Refutations* (which may be seen as closer to sophistry). There is a double movement at the foundations of thought: bringing together, then separating. We explain to very young children that apples, pears and grapes are types of fruit – they belong to a category. Does that mean that they are the same? No, they must first be separated in order to describe their differences.

From *Beyond the Pleasure Principle* (Freud, 1920) to *An Outline of Psychoanalysis* (1940 [1938]), Freud kept to one definition only of the drives:

They are of a conservative nature. . . . The aim of [Eros] is to establish ever greater unities and to preserve them thus – in short, to bind together; The aim of the [destructive instinct] is, on the contrary, to undo connections and so to destroy things. In the case of the destructive instinct, we may suppose that its final aim is to lead what is living into an inorganic state.

(1940, p. 148)

The two basic instincts are concurrent and mutually opposing. "Modifications in the proportion of the fusion between the instincts have the most tangible results" (ibid. p. 149).

In an attempt to summarise my thoughts on the question of thought in the Freudian corpus, I would say that we are faced with a constant confusion between thought and mental functioning, which overlap but differ. Ideas are needed for thinking, but they do not suffice to constitute thought. Thought requires a subject who thinks and a cathected (internal) object which reflects his "investiture".[4] If desire and the conception of the drive are indispensable, it was only, I think, after "Narcissism: An introduction", and then *Beyond the Pleasure Principle*, that Freud's work made it possible to raise the question of thought processes. This was thanks to the second drive opposition, which I assume was based in Freud's knowledge of Greek philosophy.

Four years later, the recognition of primary erotogenic masochism – which requires the delay, suspension and retention of the libido, mechanisms that I consider to be the basis of all mentalisation – and finally, "Negation" (Freud, 1925), gave us the indispensable tools. Negation is not a mere rejection, but the root of the subject. The initial "No" is a rejection that differentiates between the inside and the outside and brings into being the "I". Saying no is above all an affirmation of identity. Freud's point of departure is strictly clinical. "The content of a repressed image or idea can make its way into consciousness, on condition that it is *negated*; negation is a way of taking cognizance of what is repressed ['In the dream, it is not my mother']" (pp. 235–236). Thus, Freud, stresses how "the intellectual function is separated from the affective process" (ibid.). With the help of negation, "thinking frees itself from the restrictions of repression and enriches itself with material that is indispensable for its proper functioning" (ibid.). The operation of judgment is thus made possible by the creation of the symbol of *negation, a precondition of the independence of thought*.

On the extensions of Freud

I am not attempting to be exhaustive here and therefore will not be discussing Klein and Bion. Speaking of thought in Freud's work leads me to pay tribute to the work of André Green, which elucidated, explored and extended Freudian metapsychology. Without him, fundamental conceptions that were outlined or left incomplete would no doubt still be obscure for us today. Although it is rooted in metapsychology, Green's work is in itself of considerable importance, in particular concerning affect, narcissism and language. It not only throws light on and extends the Freudian corpus, but adds new chapters to it. Freud had said nothing about language, apart from the fact that analysis is a talking cure.

As chance, or the unconscious, would have it, I came across *Corps et affects* by Françoise Héritier and Margarita Xanthakou. Étienne Bonnot de Condillac is cited in the introduction: "Thought without signs would be restricted and unable to reach abstraction. Language is consequently a purely human invention which frees us from animality reduced to sensation, perception and a primary level of emotion" (Condillac is cited by Héritier & Xanthakou, 2004, p. 14). For Condillac, sensations and perceptions are at the origin of thought, but only language can organise it. To this point of view, Freud added the concepts of thing-presentations and word-presentations, as well as the idea that affect results from the connection between emotion and representation.

And further on, Héritier refers to an early article by António Damasio (2003), "L'esprit est modelé par le corps" (The mind is shaped by the body). Damasio shows the difference between emotions as reflex responses to stimuli and to feelings, responses that serve as formations of cerebral representations for the subject of these emotions, and what he calls the "reflexive consciousness of this feeling" which can be shared through language.

I have wondered how "the reflexive consciousness of a feeling" can be translated into psychoanalytic terms. Is it not similar to what Green calls the "self-reflexive capacity of the psyche"? For Green, affect itself lies at the roots of the self-reflexive capacity of the ego as a result of an attribution of quality to affect which permits it secondarily to acquire a "psycho-physiological function of introspection centred on the self-perception of an internal movement of the body" (see Cupa & Pirlo, 2012 and Delourmel, 2005).

This idea seems crucial to me, particularly as it coincides with the most recent views of present-day neurobiologists. During a consultation at the Paris Institute of Psychosomatics (IPSO), a young woman told me that she had not paid any attention to her somatic symptom and it was the anxiety she read in the eyes of the doctor who was examining her that suddenly made her feel physical unease and anxiety. We can easily see here the circuit through the object described by Green.

I will conclude by making a few remarks on the crucial role of language in the circuit of emotion between body, brain and mind. Psychoanalysis is a "talking cure". Green was one of the first to see the key role of language in the circuit of emotion between body, brain and mind. I am not overlooking the importance of Lacan who, with "The function of speech and language" (Lacan, 1953; see also Anzieu, 1953) known as the "Discourse of Rome", was the first to attempt to develop a theory of language in psychoanalysis; but it seems to me that he lost sight of the frame of analysis, and in particular, the circuit body/emotion/affect which Green always highlighted.

In the Freudian model of analytic treatment, the frame and the stating of the fundamental rule place the patient in an unusual experimental situation where nothing is permitted outside speech. The analysand must therefore transfer his entire mental functioning through language.

In "Le langage dans la psychanalyse", Green (1984)[5] described "a double process of transference: transference of the psychic on to speech and transference of speech on to the analyst/object" (p. 132). The conversion of the psychical apparatus into language, a source of infinite metaphorical possibilities, opens up new associative paths. However, these new associations, which convey memories, must once again pass through the body to re-find the emotion that will make this discourse living and a vehicle of change. Green writes that, in analysis, "the apparatus of language appears to be an artificial analagon of the psychical apparatus, a unifying, homogenizing and vectorizing conversion of it" (ibid.).

Indeed, for Green (1999/1973) analytic speech seeks to "take the mourning out of language" (p. 310), to make it a living discourse where the flow of associations is a mark of the return of the drive. Psychosomaticians can only confirm this idea; for what we call "operational (*opératoire*) functioning" is paradigmatic of a disembodied discourse in which neither speech nor thought are an "act of the flesh". The whole work of the psychosomatician/psychoanalyst consists in reembodying this abstract thought, cut off from images – from thing-presentations.

A double operation must therefore be conceived: if thinking is an *act of the flesh*, this act of the flesh must have been transformed into language. This transformation is a constraint that has intelligibility as its aim. However, language possesses its own self-organisation and genius. Like thought, language seeks to master statements, yet at the same time, it is a source of infinite metaphorical and associative possibilities. In analysis, the psychoanalyst looks for the infiniteness of the associative possibilities, in which the repetition compulsion is thwarted. Jean-Clause Rolland shows this with talent.[6] What I have called a "double operation" occurs in two stages: constraint and liberation, or construction and deconstruction. There is, in effect, a paradox with regard to thought in the context of the psychoanalytic treatment. The fundamental rule aims both to facilitate the deployment of thought (conversion of the drive into word-presentations) and to destabilise it. The rule of free association thus seeks to facilitate the deployment of conscious thought and its destabilisation through the irruption of the unconscious.

This paradoxicality, which plays out at different levels, no doubt contributes to the extreme difficulty in developing a true theory of thinking in psychoanalysis. It seems to me that, while we know how thought processes are formed and undone in analysis, this does not mean that psychoanalysis can or must develop its own theory of thinking.

Notes

1 "On the Resurrection of the Flesh", *The Apology*.
2 See Bollas (2007), where the author explores the interest of the notion of unconscious perception.
3 The name *Organon* does not derive from Aristotle himself, but is attributed to Dio-
genes Laertius. While Empedocles, a pre-Socratic philosopher from Agrigento,
had identified four elements – fire/air/water/earth – Aristotle, more logically,
established the series fire, air, water, earth. To the four elements, Empedocles
added "two forces" – Love, which brings together even that which is dissimilar,
and Strife, which separates what is joined.
4 The term is used by André Green (2000b) in "Primary narcissism: structure or
state", Chapter Two in *Life Narcissism, Death Narcissism*. He writes that the subject
builds his personality, thanks to this *investiture* of the object. In the same chapter,
he speaks of the "framing structure of the mother".
5 See also Green (2007), as well as the chapter "Du langage dans la psychanalyse",
in the excellent work tool by Cupa and Pirlo (2012).
6 See in Rolland (1998) the chapters "Du rêve au mot d'esprit, la fabrique de la
langue" (pp. 169–201) and "Compulsion de répétition, compulsion de représentation" (pp. 201–259); see also Rolland (2010).

References

Aisenstein, M. (2010). Les exigences de la représentation. *Revue française de psych-
analyse* 74(5): 1367–1392.
Aisenstein, M., & Dreyfus, S. (1995). De la référence aux modèles philosophiques en
psychanalyse et en psychosomatique. *Revue française de psychosomatique* 7(1):
153–172.
Anzieu, D. (1953). Fonction de la parole et du langage. In: *Psychanalyser I*, D.
Anzieu. Paris: Dunod, pp. 152–164.
Bollas, C. (2007). *The Freudian Moment*. London: Karnac.
Cupa, D & Pirlo, G. (2012). *André Green*. Paris: Presses Universitaires de France.
Damasio, A. (2003). L'esprit est modelé par le corps. In: *La Recherche 368*. Paris: Edi-
tions Sophia, pp. 70–81.
Delourmel, C. (2005). Quelques figures de la tiercéité dans l'œuvre d'André Green.
In: *Enjeux pour une psychanalyse contemporaine*, ed. F. Richard. Paris: Presses Uni-
versitaires de France, pp. 327–343.
Freud, S. (1895). *Studies on Hysteria*. *S.E.*, 2. London: Hogarth.
Freud, S. (1896). The aetiology of hysteria. *S.E.*, 3. London: Hogarth, pp. 191–221.
Freud, S. (1900). *The Interpretation of Dreams*. *S.E.*, 4–5. London: Hogarth.
Freud, S. (1905a [1890]). Psychical (or mental) treatment. *S.E.*, 7. London: Hogarth,
pp. 283–302.
Freud, S. (1905b). *Three Essays on the Theory of Sexuality*. *S.E.*, 7. London: Hogarth,
pp. 123–243.
Freud, S. (1910). *Leonardo da Vinci and a Memory of His Childhood*. *S.E.*, 11. London:
Hogarth, pp. 57–137.
Freud, S. (1911). Formulations on the Two Principles of Mental Functioning. *S.E.*,
12. London: Hogarth, pp. 218–226.
Freud, S. (1914). *On Narcissism: An Introduction*. *S.E.*, 14. London: Hogarth,
pp. 69–102.

Freud, S. (1915). *Instincts and their Vicissitudes. S.E.*, 14. London: Hogarth, pp. 109–140.

Freud, S. (1917). *A Metapsychological Supplement to the Theory of Dreams. S.E.*, 14. London: Hogarth, pp. 222–235.

Freud, S. (1920). *Beyond the Pleasure Principle. S.E.*, 18. London: Hogarth, pp. 1–64.

Freud, S. (1925). Negation. *S.E.*, 19. London: Hogarth, pp. 233–239.

Freud, S. (1940 [1938]). *An Outline of Psychoanalysis. S.E.*, 23. London: Hogarth, pp. 139–207.

Freud, S. (1950 [1895]). *Project for a Scientific Psychology. S.E.*, 1. London: Hogarth, pp. 295–397.

Green, A. (1984). Le langage dans la psychanalyse. In: *Langages: IIe Rencontre psychanalytiques d'Aix-en-Provence, 1983*, eds. A. Green, G. Diatkine, E. Jabès, et al. Paris: Les Belles Lettres, pp. 19–250.

Green, A. (1999/1973). *The Fabric of Affect in the Psychoanalytic Discourse*, trans. A. Sheridan. London: Routledge & the Institute of Psycho-Analysis.

Green, A. (2000a/1983). *Life Narcissism, Death Narcissism*, trans. Andrew Weller. London: Free Association Books.

Green, A. (2000b/1983). Primary narcissism: Structure or state. In: *Life Narcissism, Death Narcissism*. London: Free Association Books, pp. 48–90.

Green, A. (2007). Langue, parole psychanalytique et absence. *Revue française de psychanalyse* 71(5): 1461–1471.

Héritier, F., & Xanthakou, M. (2004). Retour à Condillac. In: *Corps et affects*. Paris: Odile Jacob, pp. 12–14.

Lacan, J. (1953/2005). The function and field of speech and language in psychoanalysis. In: *Écrits*, trans. Bruce Fink. New York, NY: Norton, pp. 197–268.

Rolland, J.-C. (1998). *Guérir du mal d'aimer*. Paris: Gallimard.

Rolland, J.-C. (2010). *Les yeux de l'âme*. Paris: Gallimard.

Rosenberg, B. (2003). Masochisme mortifère, masochisme gardien de vie. In: *Monograph of La Revue française de psychanalyse*. Paris: Presses Universitaires Françaises.

Tertullian (1929). *Apologeticum* (197 A.C.), trans. T. H. Bindley. Available on www.earlychurchtexts.com.

6 On the destruction of thought processes*

In September 2004, at a Colloquium at Cerisy in tribute to André Green (Richard & Uribarri, 2005), I gave a paper titled the "Échecs et destruction des processus de representation" (Aisenstein, 2005), a subject that continues to nourish my reflections. We are living in times of "social unbinding", in the terms of sociologists – of discontents in civilisation – which is increasingly conducive to learning for not thinking – to the decline of humanism. Contemporary psychoanalytic clinical practice often confronts us with patients who, in order to express themselves, need to resort to forms of acting – behavioural expressions or somatisation; in other words, we are faced with processes which short-circuit psychical elaboration. These patients do not present intrapsychic conflicts, but a state of unease and ill-being which requires immediate responses. In my view, our Western civilisation contributes to the crushing of thought and the capacity to wait and defer, thereby favouring the short path rather than the more appropriate "long path" described by Freud (1911).

We are living in a culture of fast-food, communication at the speed of lightning, and even of a demand for "fast analysis". At the same, we are at an important historical moment in which the human sciences such as neurobiology and immunology confirm the ideas of Green (1973). I am thinking, of course, of António Damasio (1994), who speaks of the "emotional brain" and emphasises the importance of affect; I am also thinking of Alain Prochiantz (1989) who accepts the role played by the subject's personal history and of fantasy in explaining the great capacity of the human genetic programme. I am also referring to the immunologist Jean-Claude Ameisen (1999), a theoretician of apoptosis – that is, of cell death – according to whom organic functions can be deeply modified through a narrative construction.

This contradiction, this paradox, faces us with the crucial question of the internal destructiveness of the human mind and of its conflict with the

* This chapter was first published in 2014 under the title "Destruction des processus de la pensée et processus de la sublimation" in the *Revue française de psychosomatique* (Sublimation), 46: 9–20.

DOI: 10.4324/9781003197652-7

life drives, which, in *An Outline of Psychoanalysis*, Freud (1940a) calls Eros: a force that binds together and aims "to establish ever greater unities" (p. 148). A few lines further on in the same text, he adds that the death drive aims to undo connections and so "to destroy things".

Binding/unbinding is related to the heart of the problem of meaning. Binding together several elements amounts to creating a meaning that can be appropriated, which gives rise to the sense of subjectivation and to thinking about oneself as a subject. Unbinding – destroying connections – amounts to annihilating meaning, which triggers mechanisms and processes of de-objectalisation and de-subjectivation, as Green has described so well.

At the Cerisy Colloquium, I focused my remarks on pathological forms of negative hallucination and on psychosomatic clinical practice (Aisenstein, 2005). I would like here to recall certain premises. The "operational (*opératoire*) states" described by the Paris School of Psychosomatics are pathognomic lines of the clinical experience of the negative. The heuristic concept of "mentalisation" introduced by the psychosomaticians of the Paris School essentially concerns processes of representation. It accounts for the capacity of the mental apparatus to bind instinctual drive excitation with networks of representation. "De-mentalisation", the most characteristic example of which is "operational thinking", can be observed in certain cases of somatic illnesses. It also appears during the transitory traumatic states that any individual may experience. To this particular type of psychopathological configuration, I would add, for my part, a third category that I have called the "clinical phenomenon of conformism" (Aisenstein, 2001).

This de-mentalisation may be understood as an anti-traumatic strategy in the interests of survival. This anti-traumatic strategy is not a classical mental defence, like, for example, delusion, but it denotes possibilities of discharge through the soma, behavioural manifestations or acting out. The obstacles standing in the way of mentalisation are linked to certain failures of hallucinatory wish-fulfilment at the beginnings of psychic life. These failures are at the origin of deficiencies in establishing auto-erotic activities and fantasy life. The notion of anti-traumatic defence, or anti-traumatic strategy, implies a struggle against anxiety and painful affects at any price. When repression and negation are no longer efficient, the subject resorts to the splitting and disavowal of reality. The concept of the negative makes it possible to reconsider de-mentalisation and the lasting, underlying operational states of somatic disorganisations from the angle of the second drive theory and of splitting.

Freud's article on splitting, written in 1938, remained unfinished. Freud seems hesitant, wondering if he is describing a new entity or such a familiar human phenomenon that it seems self-evident. He mentions a "rift in the ego that will never heal, indeed it will widen as time goes on" (Freud, 1940b, p. 296). It is important to note that such a cut is not a division between two psychic systems; it is oriented against perception and permits a non-dialectical co-existence between an affirmation and a negation.

Alongside fetishism and psychosis, such forms of splitting also seem to me to be common place in psychosomatics. I have formulated the hypothesis in connection with them that a split exists at the level of endosomatic perceptions; thus, at the very specific level of the "clinical phenomenon of conformism". I would also add a level that I define as "terrifying normality".

Adolf Eichmann appeared to be a normal man: courteous, cooperative and, apparently, in a typical state of de-mentalisation. He did not deny that he had contributed to a massive catastrophe, which he claimed he had not wanted. He seemed to be devoid of guilt, since he placed efficiency and obedience to authority above all other values. He said he had always been horrified by violence, and there is no reason to doubt it. Here is one of his replies to the chief prosecutor: "If I had been named as the head of an extermination camp at that moment, I would have killed myself . . . given my reactions . . . and what I knew at the time . . . (given that I could not imagine it), I think I would have ended my life to escape this situation".[1]

In order to be able to think about this unthinkable dimension, which nonetheless exists, I think that notions such as the desexualised cultural superego or the regression of the superego to the ego-ideal prove insufficient, unless they are considered as possible transformations of a deadly work of the negative and of a "rift in the ego that will never heal".

Wanting to think about the unthinkable may seem megalomanic. While I am convinced that we are simply craftsmen when we work with our patients, I think that, as psychoanalysts, we are inevitably confronted with cultural facts. Moreover, for Freud, psychoanalysis is a "work of culture".

In *The Future of an Illusion* (Freud, 1927), he explicit links the superego to *Kulturarbeit*. The heir of the Oedipus complex, the superego is also constituted through the work of culture. Freud places the structure of the superego in the context of a dialectic between the cultural and the intrapsychic, which culminates in drive renunciation and drive transformations. In *Civilization and its Discontents*, Freud (1930) takes up the same idea and develops it to the point of describing a "process of civilisation" implying the sacrifice of instinctual drive satisfactions in favour of a "great human community".

Drive renunciation and drive transformations are related to sublimation. I will now develop this question, which I will call "the negative of sublimation".

A negative of sublimation?

The patient of my clinical material is called Maximilian Aue. A German officer in the Waffen-SS, he was thirty-four years old in 1945, at the end of the war, and is the hero and narrator of *Les Bienveillantes* (The Benevolent), a magnificent book by Jonathan Littell (2006). The title alludes to the Eumenides, the third and last part of Aeschylus' *Oresteia*. The Eumenides are both the opposite and a transposition of the Erinyes.

Maximilian Aue is a young man, neither likeable nor dislikeable, with a very complex personality. During the nine hundred and five pages of the book, the protagonist addresses the reader and describes his mental functioning, speaking in the first person. He had been a difficult child and adolescent of a French Alsatian mother and a German father. His father, whom he had loved and idealised very much, had abandoned the family before disappearing completely when Maximilian was eight years old. The mother had remarried a few years later with a French industrialist. Maximilian hated his mother, who had been unable to keep his father. The softness of her body disgusted him; he is full of recriminations towards her, even though she was tender towards him and showered him with gifts.

But he had an incestuous passion for his twin sister. He was conscious of the situation and understood very well that his homosexuality stemmed from this family configuration. His mother had offered him a piano, which he hated. He says:

> I never really loved my mother; I even detested her. It was also partly her fault. If she had insisted, if she had been able to be strict when it was necessary, I might have been able to learn to play the piano, and that would have been a great joy, a safe refuge. . . . It's just like my male loves: the reality, I am not ashamed of saying it, is that I would no doubt have preferred to be a woman . . . a naked woman, on her back, with her legs spread, crushed under the weight of a man, clinging to him, penetrated by him and drowned in him. Instead of that I became a jurist, a security official, an SS officer, and then the director of a lace factory. It's sad, but it is like that.
>
> (Littell, 2006, p. 40, translated from the French)

Further on, we read:

> It is also true that I love a woman. Only one but more than anyone else. However, she was the one who was forbidden for me. It is quite possible that by dreaming of being a woman, by dreaming of having a woman's body, I was still looking for her, I wanted to be closer to her, I wanted to be like her, I wanted to be her. I didn't love any of the men I slept with, I used their bodies, that's all. Her love would have sufficed for life. Don't laugh: this love is probably the only good thing I have done. All this, you are probably thinking, may seem a bit strange for an officer of the *Shutzstaffel*. But why wouldn't an *SS-Obersturmbannführer* have an inner life of desires and passions like any other man?
>
> (ibid. p. 29, translated from the French)

Les Bienveillantes is a historical fresco of the war exuding terrible pessimism: wars never end because human beings carry destructiveness within themselves, and this destructiveness can take on unfathomable forms. The narrator is convincing. He is cultivated, has a doctorate in law and had wanted to study philosophy. He has a keen interest in Emmanuel Kant and literature. Michael Lermontov is one of his favourite authors. He has a musical vocation and admits to having a weakness for François Couperin and French music. He cites Tertullian and reads the Greek philosophers.

He mentions that, as a child, he was allergic to milk and dairy products. He suffers from many benign somatisations, spasmodic colitis, bouts of diarrhoea and dermatitis. In the autumn of 1941, in Kiev, he suffered from vomiting every evening, a symptom he has had ever since. During the Russian campaign, of which he gives a striking description, he started having lots of nightmares.

Maximilian Aue was sent to Simferopol in the Crimea to prepare the invasion of the Caucasus. He was assigned to the sector of investigations of ethnic minorities, where he had to study interethnic relations and the relations between minorities and the central Soviet power. He did exhaustive research based on the bibliography of ethnological sciences, and it was at this point that he met the person who was to become his only true friend: Dr. Voss, a linguist specialised in Iranian and Caucasian languages. He was passionately interested in languages and comparative phonetic systems. Concerning Voss, Maximilian writes:

> I was attracted by the relationship he had to his knowledge. The intellectuals that I had frequented were constantly developing their knowledge and their theories. . . . Voss' knowledge, however, seemed to live within him like an organism, and Voss delighted in this knowledge as he might a lover, sensually; he bathed in it, constantly discovered new aspects of it that were already present in him but of which he was not yet aware, and he took the pure pleasure of a child learning to open and close a door or to fill a bucket with sand and then to empty it; anyone who listened to him shared this pleasure.
>
> (ibid., p. 317)

One cannot better describe an associative discourse and living thought. The fascinating discussions between Voss and Aue, full of brilliant erudition, intelligence and humour give the impression that affects are circulating freely. Yet the two men are faced with other specialists, anthropologists and linguists who are subjected to pressure from the Wehrmacht to accelerate the research. They are trying to find out if a small people of mountain Caucasians, who speak a dialect similar to Iranian and practice a Muslim religion, are of Semitic origin or not. The issue at stake is obviously, should they be exterminated or not?

I would readily speak at length about this impressive book that can be approached from many angles, but I will limit myself to raising certain questions.

According to Freud, sublimation is a detour of the drive, thanks to civilisation. Maximilian and his friend Voss are caught up in an unbridled process of sublimation, which, in my view, is deadly. They seem to feel protected from the horror that surrounds them – horror that they do not deny, thanks to their clearly scientific and sublimatory interest in their mission.

As a reader, I was astonished to find I let myself be lured into the trap and "contaminated" by this deadly sublimation – if one accepts this term – to the point of forgetting, or rather setting aside, the initial subject – that is, the extermination of human beings by human beings. And yet, in the book, it is impossible to forget this dimension for a moment. We are alongside the trenches; Voss and Aue see them and speak about them constantly. Moreover, they do not agree with what is going on; they think that the final solution is a historic error. Voss feels uneasy and argues that racial anthropology is a web of falsehoods.

It seems evident to me that *Les Bienveillantes* could not have been published twenty years ago, because a change of generation was necessary. It is not the only book that deals with the attachment of man to barbarism while trying to understand its functioning from the inside. The author of *Les Bienveillantes* is thirty-eight years old, was born in New York, lives in Barcelona and worked on this book for fifteen years. His father is a historian and author of novels. In an interview with *Le Monde*, he said that he had close contact with executioners in Bosnia, Chechnya and Afghanistan and that he had witnessed genocides:

> The only way [of understanding] was to put oneself in the skin of the executioner. I had become familiar with the experience of the executioner. I had rubbed shoulders with them. I started from what I knew, that is, me, with my way of thinking about and seeing the world, telling myself that I was going to slip into the skin of a Nazi. . . . Not towards the light, but by going further into the darkness, arriving in a darkness that was even darker than the darkness at the outset.
>
> (Littell, 2007)

Why have I preferred to speak about this book and Maximilian Aue rather than psychosomatic clinical practice? I had already chosen the theme of "The destruction of thought processes" in order to tackle de-mentalisation and conformism. But reading *Les Bienveillantes* moved me deeply and shook up some of my convictions. In reality, analysts are familiar with de-mentalisation – the failure of representation and the splitting of the ego. This knowledge reassures and protects us. We can speak about de-mentalisation and the "banality of evil", as I did myself. But reading *Les Bienveillants* turns everything on its head. We are caught in a whirlwind of uncertainties, which, moreover, is the aim of the book. One might reply that it is just a book, a historical fresco, well-documented and fictional.

But, in my view, literature is a source of clinical knowledge; it is a psychic function. The amazement I felt on reading this book led me to ask myself questions.

These questionings pointed me towards the paradoxes of sublimation. Green (1999) speaks about them in Chapter Eight of *The Work of the Negative*, certain points of which I will recall briefly.

After a rigorous review of classical Freudian themes, Green refers to the text "Leonardo and the memory of his childhood" (Freud, 1910) in order to show why sublimation, as a vicissitude of the drive, implies de-sexualisation. Sexual desire is transformed into artistic creativity and hunger for knowledge – which is another way of exerting mastery and control over the object. This takes us back to the ideas set out in *Life Narcissism, Death Narcissism* (Green, 2001). De-sexualisation has as its consequence the transformation of object-libido into narcissistic libido. The superego confers more value on instinctual-drive renunciation than on instinctual-drive satisfaction. We find ourselves on the side of the ego-ideal. Moreover, all active de-sexualisation causes a reduction of the energetic level of drive fusion, which leaves the path wide open for destructiveness and unbinding. Sublimation is thus, paradoxically, on the side of the death drive, and *Life Narcissism, Death Narcissism* shows this very clearly. But how can we better understand the mechanisms of the perversion of sublimation? In other words, what is this unbinding related to?

My hypothesis is that this unbinding acts against every human element, thereby introducing a misunderstanding, or misuse, of the notion of "civilisation". Freud had clearly stated that civilisation presupposes a large human community, an idea I share. When the conception of civilisation is cut off from the human being, it can lead to an artistic idea or a dangerous ideology.

I participated recently as a psychoanalyst in a scientific meeting organised by neurologists, on the theme of the specificity of hallucinations in patients with dementia. One of the questions raised was whether the doctor/therapist should intervene at the level of the content of the hallucinatory production. Some patients had described or drawn their hallucinations. The neurologists wanted to carry out research on the basis of the hypothesis that, for a certain category of patients with dementia, hallucinations follow a gradient going from the inanimate towards the human. The first drawings showed stones, bricks and square shapes, then animals, then silhouettes and faces. Among the ten participants in the group, there was a renowned painter with whom we exchanged points of view that were as lively as they were diametrically opposed. In my view, it seems plausible that mentally deficient patients may be able to develop hallucinatory psychic activity of better quality, ranging from the most simple images and utility objects towards more complex images, such as human figures. Feeling very angry, the artist categorically defended the opposite: according to him, the quality of an image lies in its deconstruction, which goes from figuration towards the sign – that is to say, abstraction. As I was preparing an article on sublimation, I wondered if the artistic passion of this painter had not led him to forget that he was in a department of medicine whose task was to understand and care for human beings.

After this detour, I will now return to my questions. The first arises from André Green's thinking: it is conceivable that, in sublimation, unbinding occurs owing to the de-fusion of the death drive, which turns against the human element, which it attacks in particular. When used inappropriately, this "perversion" of classical sublimation, which is in the service of civilisation, establishes a process of de-objectalisation, followed by de-subjectivisation.

This question is of crucial importance. Quite apart from the problem of Nazism and other totalitarian ideologies, it seeks to account for the perverse, inhuman deviations of ideologies and of those that we encounter in our clinical work with patients caught in the trap of "death sublimations" in which art and thinking put themselves in the service of destructiveness. Even psychoanalysis can fall into the trap of ideological totalitarianisms.

In the service of life

The patient was a young female doctor of Italian origin who had come to Paris ten years earlier to pursue her specialty. She had requested an analysis after a major depressive episode following the breakdown of a relationship, which was part of a series of losses. Towards the end of the sixth year of analysis, which had been focused essentially on elaborating depressive difficulties in connection with a very intrusive maternal imago, the patient had discovered, behind the image of the idealised mother, her hatred of her dependence on her mother, who wanted to maintain her mastery by cutting her daughter off from her – a mother whom the patient was discovering once again in analysis. Laëticia had cathected her analysis to such an extent that she wondered if she would not become a psychoanalyst herself. She was attending seminars in paediatrics and had begun her specialty in child psychiatry. A year before, in spring, she had formed an intense and serious love affair, but which was also complicated because her partner lived and worked in Rome. On returning from her winter vacation, she told me at the beginning of the session that, after careful consideration, she had decided to put an end to the relationship with this man who, during the vacation, had asked her to marry him. She loved him, certainly, but for her, there was no question of leaving Paris because of her analysis with me. She said this crisply and coldly, without any affective tonality. I felt anger welling up in me, which surprised me. I did not understand what I was feeling and, while trying to stay calm, I said to her, "For me, psychoanalysis is in the service of life, and not the other way round". I was not very happy with this intervention of trivial generality, and it was only subsequently that I understood that it reflected my absolute refusal to identify with the mother, who had impeded Laëticia's autonomy. When she was an adolescent, every time she planned to go out or to make a trip, her mother would say to her, "You have better things to do, stay with me and do your homework". After the silence that followed my intervention, the patient spoke about this precise recollection.

In the countertransference, the first alarm signal was the absence of affect when the patient told me about such a serious decision. The transitory unbinding in my insight was due to the negative version of our common sublimation: psychoanalysis.

Note

1 Well after this historic trial – the first trial of genocide conducted publicly in Israel in front of one of its organisers – a trial that crystallised the collective Israeli conscience by restoring a common history at a time when Israel was building its identity by turning its back on the diaspora – a book by Sylvie Lindeperg and Annette Wieviorka (2016) was published, which described a monstrous, devious and calculating Eichmann, very different from the bland and colourless official from whom Hanna Arendt derived her notion of the "banality of evil". I believe this exists, however, even if it was not the case of Eichmann.

References

Aisenstein, M. (2001). De l'obéissance. *Libres Cahiers pour la psychanalyse* 4: 93–97.

Aisenstein, M. (2005). Échecs et destruction des processus de représentation. In: *Autour de l'oeuvre de André Green. Enjeux pour une psychanalyse contemporaine*, eds. F. Ricard, F. Uribarri. Paris: Presses Universitaires de France, pp. 193–199.

Ameisen, J.-C. (1999). *La sculpture du vivant. Le suicide cellulaire et la mort créatrice.* Paris: Seuil.

Damasio, A. (1994). *Descartes' Error. Emotion, Reason and the Human Brain.* London: Random House.

Freud, S. (1910). *Leonardo da Vinci and a Memory of his Childhood. S.E.*, 11. London: Hogarth, pp. 57–137.

Freud, S. (1911). *Formulations on the Two Principles of Mental Functioning. S.E.*, 12. London: Hogarth, pp. 218–226.

Freud, S. (1927). *The Future of an Illusion. S.E.*, 21. London: Hogarth, pp. 1–56.

Freud, S. (1930). *Civilization and its Discontents. S.E.*, 21. London: Hogarth, pp. 59–145.

Freud, S. (1940a). *An Outline of Psychoanalysis. S.E.*, 23. London: Hogarth, pp. 139–208.

Freud, S. (1940b [1938]). Splitting of the ego in the process of defence. *S.E.*, 23. London: Hogarth, pp. 271–278.

Green, A. (1973). *Le discours vivant.* Paris: Presses Universitaires de France.

Green, A. (1999/1993). *The Work of the Negative*, trans. Andrew Weller. London: Free Association Books.

Green, A. (2001/1983). *Life Narcissism, Death Narcissism*, trans. Andrew Weller. London: Free Association Books.

Lindeperg, S., & Wieviorka, A. (2016). *Le moment Eichmann*. Paris: Albin Michel.

Littell, J. (2006). *Les Bienveillantes*. Paris: Gallimard.

Littell, J. (2007). *Il faudra du temps pour expliquer ce succès*. Interview with S. Blumen-feld, Le Monde, 9 March, 2007.

Prochiantz, A. (1989). *La construction du cerveau*. Paris: Hachette.

Richard, F., & Uribarri, F. (2005). *Autour de l'œuvre de André Green. Enjeux pour une psychanalyse contemporaine*. Actes du colloque de Cerisy. Paris: Presses Universitaires de France.

7 Submission and thought*

"It was said simply, it was simple to understand". This sentence is taken from the interview of a Hutu farmer called Pancrate by the journalist Jean Hatzfeld, a reporter and writer who was passionately interested in the war in Rwanda. He went back there after the genocide of the Tutsi and stayed there for long periods in the Nyamata hills, collecting testimonies from the rare survivors. These accounts gave rise to a book titled *Life Laid Bare*, which begins as follows:

> In 1994, between eleven in the morning on Monday, April 11 and two in the afternoon Saturday, May 14, about fifty thousand Tutsis, out of a population of around fifty-nine thousand, were massacred by machete, murdered every day of the week, from nine thirty in the morning until four in the afternoon, by Hutu neighbors and militiamen, on the hills of the district of Nyamata, in Rwanda.
>
> (Hatzfeld, 2006/2000, p. 3)

This was the starting-point of that book, but also of a second, published in 2005/2003, titled *Machete Season: The Killers in Rwanda Speak*. This book focused on the Hutu killers Hatzfeld met in a prison in Nyamata.

Pancrace, Adalbert, Fulgence, and Jean were neighbours or the friends of their victims, farmers or teachers, fathers, grandfathers and young adults. These men, already convicted and without any contact with the outside world, gradually revealed their desire to give an account of these months of extermination.

Pancrace says, "The first day a messenger from the municipal judge went house to house summoning us to a meeting right away. There, the judge announced that the reason for the meeting was the killing of every Tutsi without exception. It was simply said, it was simple to understand" (ibid., p. 11).

After this first meeting, the massacre was organised.

---

* This chapter was first published in 2014 under the title "Soumission et pensée" in *La Revue française de psychanalyse*, 78(3): 671–680.

DOI: 10.4324/9781003197652-8

Adalbert recounts:

> I was a leader. . . . The first person I killed with a machete, I don't
> remember the precise details. I was helping out at the church; I laid
> on big blows, I struck home on all sides, I felt the strain of effort I was
> making, but not of death – there was no personal pain in the commo-
> tion. Therefore the true first time worth telling from a lasting memory,
> for me, is when I killed two children, April 17. For me, it was strange
> to see the children drop without any noise.
>
> (Hatzfeld, ibid., p. 25)

Jean Hatzfeld:

> It is a Rwandan custom that little boys imitate their fathers and big
> brothers, by getting behind them to copy. That is how they learn the
> agriculture of sowing and harvesting from the earliest age. That is how
> many began to prowl after the dogs, to sniff out the Tutsis and expose
> them. That is how a few children began to kill in the surrounding bush.
>
> (ibid., p. 40)

Jean Hatzfeld's book is put together in an elaborate and complex manner. It consists of short chapters which classify his dialogues with the
Hutu killers thematically: organisation, the first time, the gang, the group
spirit, women, and so on.

In the second part, the author shares his thoughts as an enlightened man
who is not a psychoanalyst but a war reporter who has experienced the raids
of ethnic cleansing in Bosnia-Herzogovina: Vukovar, the seat of Sarajevo, and
Srebenica. He has read Hannah Arendt and is familiar with her book *Eichmann in Jerusalem: A Report on the Banality of Evil* (Arendt, 1963). He draws
comparisons and makes links, but also offers some almost-clinical remarks
on the manner in which the interviews took place in the prison of Rilima.

They took place in the courtyard, face to face, on two benches, under an
acacia tree. They lasted two hours and took place in the presence of two
interpreters who noted everything in full. There was also a tape recorder.

Hatzfeld points out right away that, while the interviews with the survivors were unpredictable owing to their affects, which led to blockages,
"the killers never allow themselves to be overwhelmed by anything . . .
Each killer controls what he says in his own way . . . They speak in a
monotone" (ibid., p. 152).

Their vocabulary was often abstract and general, diluted and devoid of
images.

The killers prefer to speak about war rather than massacre or genocide,
especially when they use the pronoun "I"; they deny, they don't know,
they did nothing, they saw nothing. But as soon as Hatzfeld passes from
the informal, singular "*tu*" form to the plural "you" ("*vous*") form, the
replies became more precise: "We advanced, we hit, we cut" (ibid., p. 155).

This book is fascinating and clinical in the broad sense of the term. The clinical phenomenon recalls four different descriptions: those of Jean-Luc Donnet (1982) in "Le psychophobe", of Evelyne Kestemberg (2001), of Pierre Marty (1963), with the notion of "operational thinking" (*pensée opératoire*), and lastly, of André Green (2005) in "The central phobic position".

It is obvious, however, that all these approaches concern one and the same clinical constellation, in which we could also give a place to the secondary alexithymia described by Peter Sifneos (Sifneos & Apfel, 1979) or the "concrete thinking" described in the Anglo-Saxon psychoanalytic literature. Within this vast constellation, there are some common points: the economic dimension, the resulting impoverishment, the disembodiment of language, as if words must not evoke images – a "diluted" language, Hatzfeld writes. For my part, I would say *a language that avoids formal regression*.

On the basis these remarks, I would suggest that there is a common core: fear or panic when faced with one's own thought processes. Let me recall in passing that, in Ancient Greece, the word *panic* was a military term describing a disorganisation of the armies attributed to the music of the god Pan. Fear, then, of one's productions coming from within or returning from without; fear of one's own ideational contents or of the traumatic memories that might be activated by getting more in touch with them.

If fear, panic and even terror may be said to be one and the same thing, there are nevertheless differences: the statement "I can't think, I can't think . . ." – the nagging complaint of one of my patients, who is suffering atrociously at those moments – is quite different from that of an engineer suffering from hemorrhagic rectocolitis, who says, "I don't want to speak about my dreams".

It is different, too, from the discourse of Joseph-Désiré Bitero, the leader of the district of Nyamata and instigator of the machete massacre:

> No, I was not responsible, I was a teacher, I was a committed party member, I obeyed, I killed. In a party, a leader can't just do what he wants. Yes, I had a teaching diploma; but it wasn't for me to think about our activists' political slogans. All I had to think about was implementation.
>
> (ibid. p. 173)

This answer is strangely reminiscent of the one Adolf Eichmann gave to judge Landau and to the prosecutor who asked him what he thought his specific responsibility was in the Reich's enterprise of extermination. They may be summarised thus: "I obey; therefore I don't think".

So, whatever the forms of psychic treatment or pathologies, two distinct common denominators can be identified: the first is *thinking terrifies me*; the second is *I don't think, I obey; if I obey, I don't think*.

It is the second category that I want to discuss today.

I had dwelt on these questions in 1999 in a work group organised by *Les Libres Cahiers pour la psychanalyse (LCCP)*, volumes II and IV, which are, respectively, "Dire non" and "Les divisions de l'Être". The *LCCP* had adopted a format that I like very much. Each volume was based on a text by Freud which served as a basis for discussion; in this case it was "Negation" (Freud, 1925) for Volume II and "The splitting of the ego in the process of defence" (Freud, 1940) for Volume IV. Twelve years later, I want to return to these crucial texts.

Briefly, I would say that the text of 1925 concerns the birth of thinking. For Freud, negation is not merely a refusal but the root of the subject. Saying "No" is first and foremost an affirmation of identity: "No, that's outside me"; that's not me; it doesn't come from inside me, so "I didn't think that"; I don't want to recognise myself in that.

Freud's point of departure is strictly clinical: "The content of a repressed image or idea can make its way into consciousness, on condition that it is *negated*. Negation is a way of taking cognizance of what is repressed". No, in the dream, "it's not my mother" (Freud, 1925, p. 235, Freud's emphasis).

On the basis of this observation, Freud notes that negation makes it possible to separate "the intellectual function from the affective process". Remember that the aim of repression is the suppression of affect. Thanks to negation, "thinking frees itself from the restrictions of repression and enriches itself with material that is indispensable for its proper functioning" (ibid. p. 236).

The operation of judgement is thus made possible through the creation of the symbol of *negation, a condition of the independence of thought*. For example, "It's simple" means: no operation of negation which makes things more complex, because the establishment of the symbol of negation indicates the existence of a mental operation that is distinct from repression. The failure of this operation implies splitting and denial, which are different, of course, from negation.

"The Splitting of the ego in the process of defence" is an unfinished manuscript written in 1938. I have always found this text both troubling and moving. Freud shows that he is disconcerted. The idea that this "rift in the ego which never heals but which increases as time goes on" is the price to be paid for a successful defence by a premature ego seems strange to me.

Subjected to intense demands from the drives, the child is frightened by an experience which tells him that the consequence would be a terrible, real danger. He must choose between recognising the danger and renouncing or denying the reality.

The child's ego responds to this conflict in two opposing but valid ways. Either he denies the reality and continues as before or he recognises the danger and takes on board the anxiety caused by this reality. "This success", Freud writes, "is achieved at the price of a rift in the ego" (ibid. p. 276).

This rift, which never heals, is not a split between agencies; it signals the nondialectical coexistence of an affirmation and a negation, and *consequently the impossibility of a negative affirmation*. With the exception of fetishism, psychosis and schizophrenic dissociation – psychic organisations in which ego-splitting takes on a pathological colouring – we may wonder, as Freud does, if it does not exist in a more general way. I think it does, and I make this assumption in a paper on the clinical manifestations of obedience and conformism (Aisenstein, 2001).

This, then, is my hypothesis. I see the early splits in the ego as organising the denials which underlie submission to authority, the loss of the capacity to think in terms of "I", of subject; thus, in short, a *conformist de-mentalisation* or rather a *de-mentalising submission*.[1]

I am not so naive as to reflect merely in terms of causality, which is why it is also necessary to think about the dilution of the superego in groups as Freud (1921) emphasised in *Group Psychology and the Analysis of the Ego*.[2]

Between 1951 and 1963, Stanley Milgram, a professor of psychology in the United States, carried out a series of experiments with the aim of revealing the forms of submission to authority – a vague and disembodied authority because it was a question of "scientific authority". He gives an account of these experiments in a book published in 1974, called *Obedience to Authority: An Experimental View* (Milgram, 1974).

These experiments were remarkable and overwhelming. We can seem them filmed by Henri Verneuil in the 1979 film *I . . . comme I care*, sequences of which were shown on French television in the 1990s. Claiming that he was carrying out research on memory, Stanley Milgram asked men and women, doctoral students in the majority, to participate as "monitors". He asked them to inflict electric shocks of increasing intensity on the subjects tested. According to the protocol, the subjects tested were strapped to armchairs with electrodes attached to their arms. They had to repeat from memory lists of pairs of words. Each error was met with electric charges of increasing intensity. The electric shocks were given by an electric shock generator and a row of switches marked from 15 volts (Slight Shock) to 375 volts (Danger Severe Shock) to 450 volts "XXX" (Lethal Shock).

In fact, the subjects tested were false subjects who imitated the fear and pain following the dummy electric shocks administered by the "monitors".

Under the cover of testing the procedures of memorisation, the Milgram experiment measured the degree of submission or resistance of the "study participants" to a protocol that enacted sessions of torture, pure and simple. The large majority of the "study participants" carried out the experiments until the end without hesitating to use the strongest levels of intensity. During the experiments, a few of them hesitated but resumed again after the intervention of unknown authority figures in white coats, who "reassured them". The images in the film by Henri Verneuil are terrifying. Milgram concludes by writing that that, in certain circumstances and in the face of authority, however vague it may be, "ordinary people, devoid of all hostility, can, simply by carrying out their task, become the agents of an atrocious process of destruction".

In short, this coincides exactly with the conclusions of Hanna Arendt (1963) in *Eichmann in Jerusalem: A Report on the Banality of Evil*.

Many people will have seen the 1999 film *Un Specialiste*.[3] Following this film, Rony Brauman (1999) published *Éloge de la désobéissance*, a book that has the interest of fostering reflection on the *verbatim* answers of Eichmann: he presents himself as an ordinary man, an involuntary agent of a destruction that he had not wanted. He does not feel guilty because he places obedience above all other values. Throughout these archives, it emerges that he never had the idea to say no to authority.

Whether it is a Hutu farmer or an engineer like Eichmann or a philosopher like Heidegger, the picture remains the same.

For me, it is a matter of seeing a bit more clearly into the inability brought about by certain circumstances to "affirm oneself negatively". I am borrowing this expression from J.B. Pontalis, who sees Melville's *Bartleby* (1853) as the hero of "negative affirmation".[4]

> *"I would prefer not to"*: can one render in another language than Bartleby's this sort of oxymoron that I would call a negative affirmation? A no that is expressed in a listless voice but with incredible insistence, an implacable but always calm firmness, a no that has the softness of a consenting yes, a refusal to give way to any demand, whether it be reasonable, understanding, benevolent or even affectionate. Bartleby is uncompromising, his resistance is radical.
>
> (Pontalis, 2000, p. 12)

I think Pontalis is right; it is less a matter of saying no than of affirming oneself negatively in relation to a group or authority. It is an affirmation of identity – Freud's "no, this is outside me" – which, in traumatic circumstances due to excess excitation, seems not to find expression. What are the reasons for this?

We can imagine a de-mentalisation due to the subject's inability to bind excitation (Fain, 1991). Recourse to the notion of "early splitting of the ego" seems interesting to me here insofar as this splitting of the ego underpins denial and paves the way for a "shared denial". This notion of Michel Fain is rooted in his interest for the individual psychic movements linked to the group and the community. Defined in *Le Désir de l'interprète* (Fain, 1982), it often serves to reinforce personal denials and probably "early rifts in the ego", which are always ready to grow bigger, as Freud (1940) writes.

There are many other ways of thinking about this "de-mentalising submission". I will just mention one of them: the creation of the false-self as described by Winnicott, which I see as a sort of "early submission for the sake of survival".

These are crucial questions and they need to be opened up and explored rather than closed. Recognising the banality of evil, the fact that, under certain circumstances, nine out of ten of us are capable of becoming executioners is not an acceptable clinical observation if it does not lead to deeper reflection.

In an article titled "Éloge de la nuance", Geneviève Welsch Jouve (2005) warns us against any form of banalisation that amounts to justification or resignation. The idea of "positive disobedience" is not a new one; it is worth recalling that Henri David Thoreau (1849) wrote a text called "Civil Disobedience", which was to influence Ghandi and the massive resistance of Indians, but also Martin Luther King and others. The idea is clear: the right to refuse is justified; first we are human beings, then subjects of a State. The right exists to refuse submission to a government that has gone adrift.

This links up with the ideas put forward by Arendt (1972), but for her, civil disobedience should be a feature of organised minorities united by common judgements and not by shared interests.

Thoreau and Arendt lead me to return to the question of groups and crowds already present in Freud and Fain.

In the later experiments constantly refined by Milgram, it turned out that the presence of a "monitor" of some sort facilitated submission to instructions. "Testers" who were left alone rebelled sooner and in greater numbers.

For psychoanalysts, this can only be a "transference in the form of a delegation of thought" on to an object, even an anonymous object. This brings us back to the proposition: thinking is dangerous and painful; in other words, not thinking is comfortable. But a transference object is needed. It is probable that those amongst our colleagues who have experience of group psychoanalysis could help us to explore these questions more thoroughly.

Finally, I will say a few words about what I call the "strange submission to psychoanalytic authority".

On more than one occasion, I have had to remind patients that analysis is in the service of life and not the other way round.

A man who was about fifty years old wanted to do an analysis five times a week because he had already done a long psychoanalysis and he thought that "five sessions was the best setting". I had to negotiate with him to impose a face-to-face therapy once a week, which was much more appropriate for him.

Another man told me how a year of analysis during which he had dragged himself to four sessions a week, in spite of the fact that he was undergoing a heavy treatment of chemotherapy at the time, had been a real ordeal, yet he insisted that "one mustn't miss one's sessions".

In all such cases, I would say that it is a misuse of psychoanalysis, where the idea of an idealised, disembodied and normative psychoanalysis opposes the process of the analysis.

In the course of a supervision, it often happens that the senior analyst is obliged to point out to the trainee that there are cases or moments when it is necessary to forget the precepts recommended by "classical analysis", and to refrain from interpreting the transference, for example. It is a matter of helping them to see that, even if we work with a model that we have incorporated, this model is not always applicable as such; and finally, that a rigorous approach must be combined with tact and flexibility so that the internalisation of the model does not amount to a submission to rules, since this always implies a risk of not thinking.

To conclude

"Desire, pain and thought" was my title. I realise as I am coming to the end of this book that I have followed a different order: pain, desire, thought and its vicissitudes.

Is this because I attribute pain with a teleological function?

Like Jean-Claude-Rolland, I believe that the pain produced by the earliest infantile experiences tends to be anaesthetised, is not "lived", and thus gives rise to inexorable repetitions which engender opaque pain. "Opaque" because it is devoid of an object and therefore of meaning. Psychoanalytic work has the task of awakening this pain and of obliging the subject to experience it so that it becomes a living source of representations.

Freud regarded anaesthesia as a cause of melancholia.

From the very beginning of a human being's life, it is probable that there is pain that is not experienced and that is incomprehensible for the mental apparatus of a new-born infant who does not have the words to express it. Who has not seen a "happy" infant surrounded with love suddenly begin to writhe and struggle, as if prey to inexpressible suffering?

In addition, he must survive; he is hungry and thirsty. Thanks to the mother and her psychic work which contains this suffering, the vital need is transformed into desire.

Only desire can give birth to the activity of thought – the pleasure and inalienable privilege of man.

But thinking is also painful and sometimes dangerous, since thinking means existing as a subject, differentiating oneself from others with all the internal, but also external and political, risks that this may entail.

In the last chapter on the destruction of thought processes, I argued that their origin is rooted either in fear of one's own representations or in what I have called "de-mentalising submission" to the environment.

It seems to me to be crucial today to be attentive to the various forms of the destruction of thought processes; for, while this affects the individual, the consequences are even more serious when it concerns the masses.

Thinking can hurt, put us in danger, but thinking is living. Living and thinking are one and the same thing.

Notes

1 In an article published in 2010 in *The International Journal of Psychoanalysis* with Claude Smadja, I established a link between the regression of the superego in groups, as described by Freud, and a regression to the ideal ego in the case of de-mentalisation following a traumatic inflow of stimuli (Aisenstein & Smadja, 2010).

2 Christian Delourmel has pointed out to me the similarity between this notion and the "subjectal unbinding" described by Green (1999) in *The Work of the Negative*.

3 Directed by Eyal Sivan on the basis of video archives of Eichmann's trial.
4 Among the heroes of negative affirmation, we can think of the tragic destiny of Ignace Philippe Semmelweis, who opposed the medical community of his time desperately.

References

Aisenstein, M. (2001). De l'obéissance. *Libres cahiers pour la psychanalyse* 4: 93–97.
Aisenstein, M., & Smadja, C. (2010). The conceptual framework of the Paris School of Psychosomatics: A clinical psychoanalytic approach to oncology. *International Journal of psychoanalysis* 91: 621–640.
Arendt, H. (1963). *Eichmann in Jerusalem: A Report on the Banality of Evil*. New York: The Viking Press.
Arendt, H. (1972). *Civil Disobedience in Crises of the Republic*. New York: Harvest Pocket Book.
Brauman, R. (1999). *Éloge de la désobéissance. A propos d'un "spécialiste": Adolf Eichmann*. Paris: Le Pommier.
Donnet, J.-L. (1982). Le psychophobe. *Nouvelle Revue de psychanalyse* 25: 199–214.
Fain, M. (1982). *Le Désir de l'interprète*. Paris: Aubier Montaigne.
Fain, M. (1991). Préambule à une étude métapsychologique de la vie opératoire. *Revue française de psychosomatique* 1(1): 59–80.
Freud, S. (1921). *Group Psychology and the Analysis of the Ego. S.E.*, 18. London: Hogarth, pp. 65–143.
Freud, S. (1925). Negation. *S.E.*, 19. London: Hogarth, pp. 233–239.
Freud, S. (1940 [1938]). Splitting of the ego in the process of defence. *S.E.*, 23. London: Hogarth, pp. 271–278.
Green, A. (1999/1993). *The Work of the Negative*, trans. Andrew Weller. London: Free Association Books.
Green, A. (2005/2000). The central phobic position: A new formulation of the free association method. In: *Psychoanalysis: A Paradigm for Clinical Thinking*. London: Free Association Books, pp. 133–168.
Hatzfeld, J. (2000). *Dans le Nu de la Vie, Récit des Marais Rwandais*. Paris: Seuil.
Hatzfeld, J. (2003). *Une Saison de machettes*. Paris: Seuil.
Kestemberg, E. (2001). De la phobie du fonctionnement mental. In: *La psychose froide*. Paris: Presses Universitaires de France, pp. 215–221.
Marty, P., de M'Uzan, M., & David, C. (1963). *L'investigation psychosomatique*. Paris: Presses universitaires de France.
Milgram, S. (1974). *Obedience to Authority: An Experimental View*. New York: Harper and Row.
Pontalis, J.-B. (2000). L'affirmation négative. *Libres Cahiers pour la psychanalyse* 2(2): 11–18. Available on www.cairn.info/revue-libres-cahiers-pour-la-psychanalyse-2000-2-page-II.htm.
Sifneos, P., & Apfel, R. J. (1979). Alexithymia: Concept and measurement. *Psychotherapy and Psychosomatics* 32: 180–190.
Thoreau, H. D. (1849). Civil disobedience. In: *Aesthetic Papers*, ed. Elizabeth P. Peabody. Boston and New York: The Editor and G. P. Putnam, pp. 189–211.
Welsch Jouve, G. (2005). Éloge de la nuance. *Psychiatrie française* 36(2): 103–123.

Annex

On primary erotogenic masochism: an imaginary dialogue with Benno Rosenberg*

Michel Fain

In 1963/1964, the morning session of a Congress had been devoted to psychosomatics. At the time, the Paris School defended the idea that the self-destruction that was observable in somatic disorders went hand in hand with a deficiency in the manifestations usually linked to masochistic cathexes, an idea that was very controversial at the time; in other words, no one had in mind the views since elaborated by Benno Rosenberg. He emphasises the culmination of the mutation of Freud's meta-psychological views represented by the article of 1924 on masochism – a culmination that opens up interesting paths of research.

Benno Rosenberg (2003) points out that, until 1920, masochism was just one path of libidinal satisfaction among others; after then, it became essentially a means of not satisfying the death drive. Due to its texture, this sentence evokes the mythical description made by Freud of the emergence of life: certain events create the conditions required for the appearance of the phenomenon of life, a creation that leads ipso facto to an inverse movement aimed at re-establishing the earlier state. Freud adds that the opposite tendency succeeded in re-establishing the inorganic state until this new phenomenon – the pleasure of suffering – appeared, which, as Benno Rosenberg would say, is the guardian of life.

Benno Rosenberg's affirmation, "masochism was just one path of libidinal satisfaction among others", merits discussion: it could, under certain conditions, lead to orgasm, or to discharge, just like the auto-erotic activities of children which are almost all underpinned by sado-masochistic fantasies.

However, and this is already a difference, the sado-masochism of the future pervert relies more on behaviour. The same is true in the failure-neurosis. Regarding these solutions, Benno Rosenberg adds, "It had become essentially the means of not satisfying the death drive" (ibid.). Is this evolution, which needs to be clarified, moreover, essential or different? It does not replace the occasional or permanent pervert. Is this "evolution" not

---

* This chapter was first published in 2000 under the title "À propos du masochisme érogène primaire. Dialogue imaginaire avec Benno Rosenberg" in M. Aisenstein, *Psychanalystes d'aujourd'hui*, Paris, Presses Universitaires de France.

also related to the evolution of Freud's theories – an evolution, as Benno Rosenberg emphasises, that was the result of observing silent resistances to analysis – resistances motivated by a "need for self-punishment"?

Thus, the adverb "essentially" is also related to the practice of analysis, and since he points out that this expression of masochism is also experienced as a guardian of life, we can understand that it can underpin powerful resistances.

What is going on during these analyses where what dominates is commonly called a "negative therapeutic reaction"? The material brought by the patient allows us initially to highlight the unconscious manifestations and the blockage of their elaborations; a particularly distressing result of this is that the material that had made these interpretations possible disappears. The analytic situation becomes the seat of a crude expression of the drives: the analyst's interpretative activity results in an impoverishment of the material brought by the patient, who denies that he derives pleasure from this result. In fact, the empty-headedness displayed by the patient denies that his head is full of precious pain, a plenitude onto which castration anxiety has been displaced.

The hypothesis concerning the genesis of this state envisages a common disorder: although a painful lack of satisfaction usually finds its compromise via hallucinatory wish-fulfilment, the latter fails here and the excitation only finds its solution in painful experience – restrained experience.

I will digress for a moment in this connection: if the death drive has the aim, among others, of suppressing sensibility to excitation by attacking both the exciting agent and the part that is excited (hence its role, emphasised by André Green, in the genesis of the stimulus barrier systems), its propensity for maintaining repetition is exhausting and collaborates in a collusion between the death drive and the traumatic element. This addition of de-structuring effects constitutes, to my mind, what Pierre Marty described as movements of death, similar, in fact, to what Benno Rosenberg describes as "deadly masochism".

Thus, an interpretation of the adverb "essentially", appearing in the quotation of a sentence of Benno Rosenberg, leads us to the problem which, after the psychosomatic practitioners, has mobilised the attention of many colleagues; namely, of un-representability. In the case of a negative reaction to analysis, this un-representability could be substituted positively by a valuable and concealed painful tension. Anyone who says "un-representability" is underlining a topographical problem: what has become of the memory traces? Agenesis or erasure? "[It] has become essentially the means of the non-satisfaction of the death drive", says Benno Rosenberg, speaking of erotogenic masochism. This statement contains a condensation which confers satisfaction on the drive; this is not a classical position, since the drive reaches its aim either directly or by means of substitution, the satisfaction being located conflictually (or not) in the ego. Would it be any different for the death drive?

According to Freud, it is the trace at the heart of all living matter of a time when any means of registration was absent, a time that can only be conceived as absolute darkness – a complete non-memory. An illuminated dark-room would represent the first pain, a flickering flame in danger from the outset of disappearing totally into obscurity. Would castration then be situated prior to the birth of any drive charged with life? The latter, always in danger, would include erasure organically in its structure.

These aspects did not escape Benno Rosenberg. In his monograph, an entire section of the last chapter is devoted to the interactions of the two drives in historicity. He writes that a relatively successful drive fusion renders the permanence of the past active and indelible. The question of the fate of memory traces during important regressions has often been raised. Now, regressions oriented towards anachronic objects become indistinguishable in their movement from the drives. The unbound portion of the death drive tries to recreate obscurity where the traces were located: in such a case, the erasure of the traces is merely one of the forms of the manifestation of ambivalence towards objects. The moral pain that commonly accompanies these regressions, pain that appears particularly acutely when a reminder from the outside is perceived of what the ego was before the regression, is thus a form of memory of the erased traces.

These speculations lead us back to the sentence cited at the beginning of this paper in 1924: "Masochism was one path of libidinal satisfaction among others"; in other words, a part-instinct organically linked to sadism, whose existence revealed the appearance of an active object.

Following Benno Rosenberg, we can add that masochism contains within itself another path that can escape elaboration. By saying that, in such a case, primary masochism goes from the subject to the subject and is a way of doing without the object, the author is emphasising the potential for splitting that it contains. It is difficult, therefore, to find a particular somatic point of attachment for it, whereas classical sado-masochism makes extensive use of sensory motricity; in other words, it is difficult to assign it an erogenous zone. In fact, situating primary masochism at the heart of living matter is a way of not situating it. Yet, in *Beyond the Pleasure Principle*, Freud (1920) had already pointed out that the suffering linked to an injury, whose boundaries are narcissistically anti-cathected, was at the origin of the economy of traumatic neurosis. Could this non-localised primary masochism be a guardian of life? Studies in psychosomatics have made the assumption that mentalised conflict is a safeguard for the body. In other words, primary masochism is only really a safeguard for life if it is localised in a precise territory unattached to major organic function (it seems to me that this point of view is close to that developed some time ago now by Jean Laplanche in connection with auto-erotism). I therefore tend to think that primary masochism only has a function as a guardian of life to the extent that it manifests itself through the body in places where organ pleasure tends to impose itself on what is functional. The notion of self-preservation in the first stages of psychoanalysis only acquired this name with the simultaneous idea of a danger menacing the subject if he makes use of the excitation of his erogenous zones; it is correlative with the worried message of the mother witnessing the auto-erotic manifestations of her child.

In my view, it is a mistake to confuse narcissistic and auto-erotic; even if, objectively, the conflict between them is in the service of conservation, this service is only ensured if there is a subjective conflict. It is possible to imagine that, initially, masochism finds satisfaction in excitation whose erotic dimension based on non-discharge leads to double suffering, one form of which is linked to jouissance. The other consequence of the observation of the very existence of this excitation is mental suffering that does not take into account the fact that this conflict that results from it, and to which it bears witness, is a safeguard for psychosomatic functioning.

The primal jouissance of the subject by the subject led Rosenberg to offer one of the most original and convincing descriptions of the weight of primary masochism in the vicissitudes and source of the drive. And yet, if this primary masochism was merely a residue of the death drive, persisting after the subject had got rid of the death drive – notably, in the form of non-erotic sadism – would it not lose its value as a fixation point – in other words, its attractive potentiality in regressions?

"Instincts and their vicissitudes" (Freud, 1915) describes the "double reversal" (i.e. turning round upon the subject's own self and reversal into its opposite) which includes the satisfaction of the object in the history of the drive, thanks to the second reversal which opens out on to the subject's passivity as a source of enjoyment. Freud perceives a narcissistic satisfaction in this outcome; in other words, a compromise solution between the anaclitic object-choices described in 1914 and narcissistic object-choices. After the ideas emitted in 1924 on the economic aspects of masochism, did Freud not substitute a return to primary masochism for a return towards the narcissism of 1915? This substitution is confirmed by Benno Rosenberg when he underlines the cathexis of the subject by the subject in the course of this primitive phenomenon. If the double reversal is accomplished sufficiently, it confers on secondary masochism the value of a compromise between the obligation to evacuate the death drive into the outside and the aspiration of the ego to maintain a sexualised retention. The pleasure of the masochist is nourished by the sadism which he knows how to provoke – a view expressed a long time ago already by Bela Grunberger. It is important to remember that the description of this mechanism of provocation of the superego by the ego prevails in failure-neurosis. This mechanism implies a re-sexualisation of the superego; that is, a rebinding of the death drive which the said superego had stocked with libido that as a result becomes erotic again. The superego loses here its anti-incestuous function.

Can it not be said, then, that the valency "guardian of life" of primary masochism is transferred, in the course of a good enough evolution, onto the passivity which permits the compromise establishing secondary masochism – the passivity that plays such an important role, by its absence, in the genesis of the biological bedrock?

Is it not paradoxical to find that the main reasons for the failures of psychoanalytic treatments are, on the one hand, the negative therapeutic reaction – a reaction whose origin lies in the existence of a masochism that is all the more operative in that it is unconscious – and, on the other, the refusal to recognise the pleasure linked to the passivity in which the masochism remains unaccomplished?

In fact, clinical experience does not always confirm the existence of repressed passivity; all too often, bad, overexciting conditions have prevented pleasant passivity from being established. Only the absence of this experience is registered in the mind. In such cases, only activity will be valued and phallic narcissism will infiltrate the ego ideal. I would say that, in people who are sufficiently balanced, narcissistic exaltation is easily transformed into masochistic provocation. Freud told us, did he not, that very often, when he felt proud of his genius, he found himself the following night in a chemistry laboratory – a place where he had experimented with cocaine and experienced failure? In other words, the feeling of merging with the ideal is retroactively generative of latent thoughts full of masochistic desire.

It was these observations, generally made in connection with somatic patients, that led me to speak of incomplete masochism. The incompletion relates to the passive position made inaccessible by early traumatic experiences; the compulsion to repeat then becomes the particular form of masochistic seduction that is active provocation. It is said of these individuals who suffer from such incompletion that they are aggressive. This is why this antecedent is frequently found in psychopaths. The boundary between neurosis and psychosis is situated within this perspective, which is why, it seems to me, paranoiacs are not masochistic. They suffer, moreover, without deriving enjoyment from this lack.

M.F.

References

Freud, S. (1915). *Instincts and their Vicissitudes*. S.E., 14. London: Hogarth, pp. 109–140.
Freud, S. (1920). *Beyond the Pleasure Principle*. S.E., 18. London: Hogarth, pp. 1–64.
Rosenberg, B. (2003). Masochisme mortifère, masochisme gardien de la vie. In: *Monographie de la Revue française de psychanalyse*. Paris: Presses Universitaires de France.

Index

For Product Safety Concerns and Information please contact our EU
representative GPSR@taylorandfrancis.com
Taylor & Francis Verlag GmbH, Kaufingerstraße 24, 80331 München, Germany

www.ingramcontent.com/pod-product-compliance
Lightning Source LLC
Chambersburg PA
CBHW050617280326
41932CB00016B/3083